Clinical Assessment Workbook
for
Communication Sciences and Disorders

Clinical Assessment Workbook for Communication Sciences and Disorders

Georgia Hambrecht, PhD, CCC-SLP
Tracie Rice, AuD, CCC-A

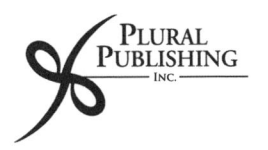

PLURAL PUBLISHING, INC.

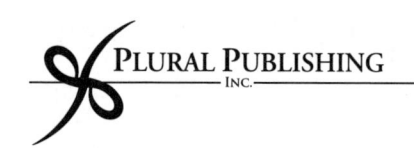

5521 Ruffin Road
San Diego, CA 92123

e-mail: information@pluralpublishing.com
Web site: http://www.pluralpublishing.com

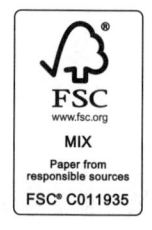

Copyright © 2020 by Plural Publishing, Inc.

Typeset in 11/14 Stone Informal by Achorn International
Printed in the United States of America by McNaughton & Gunn, Inc.

All rights, including that of translation, reserved. No part of this publication may be reproduced, stored in a retrieval system, or transmitted in any form or by any means, electronic, mechanical, recording, or otherwise, including photocopying, recording, taping, Web distribution, or information storage and retrieval systems without the prior written consent of the publisher.

For permission to use material from this text, contact us by
Telephone: (866) 758-7251
Fax: (888) 758-7255
e-mail: permissions@pluralpublishing.com

Every attempt has been made to contact the copyright holders for material originally printed in another source. If any have been inadvertently overlooked, the publishers will gladly make the necessary arrangements at the first opportunity.

Library of Congress Cataloging-in-Publication Data:
ISBN-13: 978-1-63550-034-9
ISBN-10: 1-63550-034-6

Contents

Preface	vii
Acknowledgments	ix
Reviewers	xi
Chapter 1. Introduction to Assessment	1
Chapter 2. Referrals	9
Chapter 3. Intake and Interview	19
Chapter 4. Oral-Facial Examinations	31
Chapter 5. Standardized Testing	43
Chapter 6. Statistical Basis	53
Chapter 7. Dynamic Assessment	61
Chapter 8. Observation	69
Chapter 9. Synthesizing Information	81
Chapter 10. Report Writing	91
Chapter 11. Ongoing Assessment	105
Chapter 12. Hearing Assessment	115
Chapter 13. Billing	125
Chapter 14. Insurance	137
Chapter 15. Speech Sound Disorders	149
Chapter 16. Voice Assessment	159
Chapter 17. Fluency Assessment	167
Chapter 18. Dysphagia Assessment	177
Chapter 19. Language/Literacy in Children	187
Chapter 20. Adult Language Assessment	197
Chapter 21. Cognitive Assessment	207
Chapter 22. Social Communication Assessment	217
Chapter 23. Communication Modalities	229
Chapter 24. Final Thoughts	239
Index	*295*

Preface

This workbook follows a who, what, why, when, where, how format in order to provide a clear and familiar structure for learning. In keeping with that premise, the introduction is organized in a like fashion.

Who: The authors, who find the process of answering clinically relevant questions an exciting and challenging endeavor, bring their knowledge and experience as clinicians, clinical supervisors, and instructors in Communication Science and Disorders (CSD) into each chapter. The workbook is aimed at helping the advanced undergraduate and beginning graduate student better prepare for his/her role in the assessment process through interacting with the information provided in the text.

What: Assessment is about discovering answers to clinically relevant questions through a variety of structured and unstructured means. The earlier chapters provide a broad-based look at components that are common across assessments, while the latter chapters examine specifics—speech, language, hearing, and swallowing assessment procedures.

Why: The assessment process is multifaceted and can be daunting for the learner. This workbook provides information and activities to help prepare the student for his/her upcoming role in clinical assessment.

When: This workbook builds on the foundational knowledge gained through the normal process- and disorder-related classes found in the undergraduate CSD curriculum. It is designed to be used to prepare the student for his/her entry into assessment practices.

Where: The book is appropriate as part of a methods, clinical practicum, and/or assessment class. It can also be useful as an individual tool for review and application.

How: The workbook provides evidence- and experienced-based information, highlights important terms, presents activities to promote understanding with the answers provided to encourage immediate self-correction, and challenges the learner to consider thoughtful applications.

Acknowledgments

The authors would like to acknowledge the following individuals for their help with manuscript editing and/or sample assessment examples: A. G. Bradshaw, D. E. Carter, R. A. Cox, A. D. Frady, N. T. Greenway, E. E. Lait, A. N. Manz, K. L. McDonald-Coxen, T. D. McKinney, and M. E. Momphard. Your help was truly appreciated.

Reviewers

Plural Publishing, Inc. and the authors would like to thank the following reviewers for taking the time to provide their valuable feedback during the development process:

Sandra R. Ciocci, PhD, CCC-SLP
Professor
Bridgewater State University
Bridgewater, Massachusetts

Keri Parchman-Gonzalez, MA, CCC-SLP
Clinical Assistant Professor
The University of Texas Rio Grande Valley
Edinburg, Texas

Deborah Rainer, MS, CCC-SLP
Clinical Coordinator/Senior Lecturer
Baylor University
Waco, Texas

Heather L. Thompson, PhD, CCC-SLP
Assistant Professor, SLPA Program Coordinator
California State University, Sacramento
Sacramento, California

Rosalie Marder Unterman, PhD, CCC-SLP
Associate Professor/Clinical Director
Touro College Graduate Program in Speech-Language Pathology
Brooklyn, New York

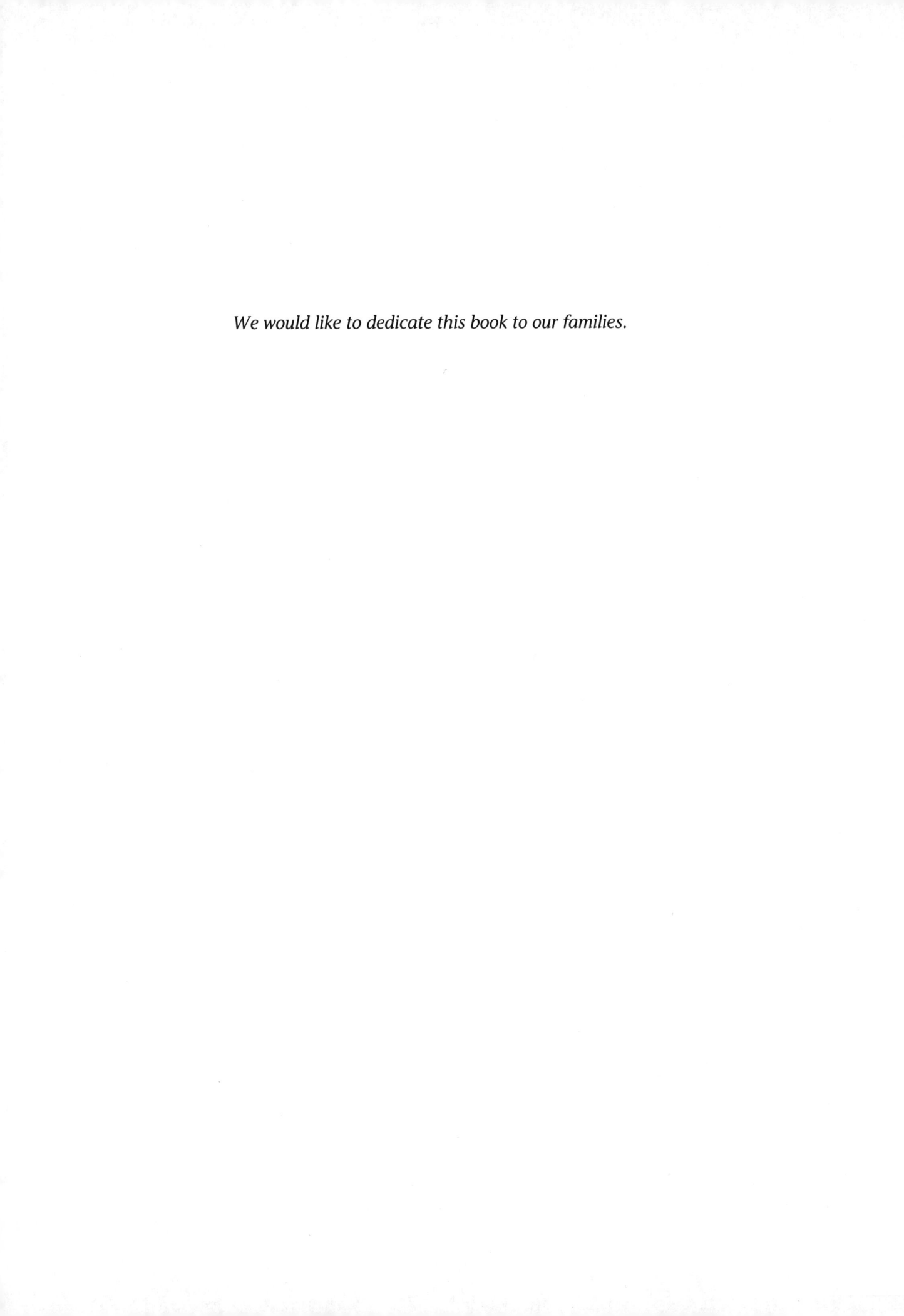

We would like to dedicate this book to our families.

CHAPTER 1

Introduction to Assessment

Who

Several people play an important role in completing an assessment. Both the client who is being evaluated and the clinician who is planning, executing, and reporting the results are central to any evaluation. Others are also involved as providers of information during the assessment or receivers of the information following the assessment (e.g., parents, teachers, doctors, and other team members).

What

Evaluations (initial or ongoing determination for eligibility) and assessments (initial and ongoing process of identification of skills) are aimed at finding the answer to one or more clinical questions (American Speech-Language-Hearing Association, n.d.; Kratcoski, 1998). Unique information is gathered depending on the question asked (Olswang & Bain, 1994; Westby, Stevens Dominguez, & Oetter, 1996). Some of the questions clinicians are asked to answer include

- Is there a need for testing?
- How does the individual's skills compare to a peer group?
- Is the client developing typically?
- Does the individual qualify for services?
- What is the present level of functioning?
- Are academics or social relationships being negatively impacted?
- What techniques will work best for remediating the errors?
- What level is the appropriate one to treat?
- What targets should be addressed?
- Is progress being made?
- Is the change a result of the remediation being provided?
- Should the client be dismissed from therapy?

With so many varied questions, which will need to be addressed at some point in your practice, it follows that there are many procedures that you will need to understand and know how to administer, interpret, and report.

Why

Communication is a vital part of people's lives. Your role as a clinician is to determine if a communication disorder exists, the extent/severity of that disorder, and recommendations for treatment or referral. There will be some procedures you will use that must be done in a very prescribed fashion. These approaches are termed static assessments and include norm referenced/standardized tests and developmental scales. Giving, scoring, and reporting on standardized tests requires precision and compliance to the administration procedures presented in the test's manual so you can compare your client to others of a similar age and gain a perspective of how he/she compares to the normative sample. There are other procedures, which determine a strategy that works for a client or determine what effect situations or partners have on the communication profile, that are better determined through a conversation, a planned/structured interaction between the client and the diagnostician, and/or observation of natural interactions. These types of assessments are termed dynamic assessment. Through static and dynamic assessments, you identify, describe, and recommend next steps.

When

When an assessment is given will depend on the questions you are trying to answer. Screenings, often a quick pass/fail procedure to identify whether a potential client needs a full assessment, are the earliest kind of evaluation. Diagnostic evaluations, usually involving norm referenced tests to determine the specific type, extent, and severity of the communication problem, are completed after a screening and prior to enrollment. Often, a block of time is set aside for this purpose. Baseline and dynamic assessments, which involve gathering information to make decisions on the specifics needed for treatment planning, may be a part of the diagnostic evaluation time block or may occur early in a scheduled treatment session. Ongoing assessment, the regular gathering of information on treatment progress, occurs throughout the remediation process. In the school setting, one-year Individualized Educational Plans (IEP) or three-year reevaluations are done at the prescribed time interval.

Where

Where the evaluation takes place is also dependent on the questions being addressed. A quiet testing room, the home, the school, the hospital room, a lab, or an informal meeting place may all be places where static and/or dynamic assessment information is gathered.

How

The way to assess will unfold in the chapters to come. It is a combination of using your knowledge, attending to the details, and caring about your client to make ethical decisions in planning, performing, and reporting assessment information.

Top 10 Terms

Baseline

Clinical questions

Developmental scales or tables

Dynamic assessment

Norm referenced/standardized test

Observation

Ongoing data collection

Screening

Static assessment

Structured interactions

Chapter Tips

1. Remember, the question or questions to be answered are driving your assessment efforts. When planning an assessment, first know what you are trying to discover and then select the procedures you will use.

2. When completing relevant paperwork (e.g., initial report, session notes or documentation, IEP forms, or progress reports), make sure it conveys information that answers the questions that are to be addressed.

3. A combination of assessment tools is used to address the assessment questions. Always incorporate a look at actual communication interactions rather than merely relying on segmented test results.

Activity

1–1. Some diagnostic procedures provide information for all the clinical questions you need to answer. Interviews and observations/conversational samples are two procedures used to address many questions. Other procedures are linked more clearly to a specific question. The following are seven questions a clinician may need to answer. Write the name of the procedure from the "Procedure

Bank" following the questions that is **most closely linked** to the question asked. A procedure will only be used once and some procedures will not be used at all.

1. _____ Is the client meeting developmental milestones?
2. _____ What techniques will work best for remediating the errors?
3. _____ How does the individual's skills compare to a sample of same-aged peers?
4. _____ I did not get enough information from the standardized test—how does the client perform on specific tasks I have arranged?
5. _____ Is there a need for testing?
6. _____ Is progress being made?
7. _____ What accuracy percentage should I set as my objective target?

Procedure Bank—select from the following procedures to fill in the blanks

Screening

Norm references/standardized test

Developmental scales or tables

Dynamic assessment

Observation

Conversational sample

Ongoing data collection

Baseline

Structured interactions

Answers to Activity

1–1

1. Developmental scales or tables
2. Dynamic assessment
3. Norm references/standardized test
4. Structured interactions
5. Screening
6. Ongoing data collection
7. Baseline

Wrap-Up

1. The authors noted that interviews and observations/conversational samples are two procedures used across many questions. Select three of the questions from the activity section of this chapter and **describe how interviews and observations/conversational samples could contribute** important information to answer the question.

   Question # ____
       Interviews:

       Observations/conversations:

   Question # ____
       Interviews:

       Observations/conversations:

   Question # ____
       Interviews:

       Observations/conversations:

2. Select three of the questions from the activity section of this chapter and identify **where** you think the best place would be to carry out the assessment to answer the question.

   Question # ____

   _____

   _____

   Question # ____

   _____

   _____

   Question # ____

   _____

   _____

3. An excellent way to review information is to compare (identifying how things are the same) and contrast (identifying how things are different) terms or concepts. Complete Table 1–1 by identifying at least 2 important ways the specified terms are the same and different.

Table 1–1. Terms and Concepts. Complete the Table with Ways That the Concepts Are the Same and Different.

Item	Terms or Concepts	Important Ways They Are the Same	Important Ways They Are Different
A.	Screening test *versus* Diagnostic test	1. 2.	1. 2.
B.	Formal testing *versus* Informal testing	1. 2.	1. 2.
C.	Dynamic testing *versus* Static testing	1. 2.	1. 2.
D.	Structured interaction *versus* Observation	1. 2.	1. 2.

continues

Table 1.1 (*continued*)

Item	Terms or Concepts	Important Ways They Are the Same	Important Ways They Are Different
E.	Assessing in a natural environment *versus* Assessing in a clinical environment	1. 2.	1. 2.
F.	Initial assessment information *versus* Ongoing data collection	1. 2.	1. 2.
G.	Ongoing data collection *versus* Baseline data collection	1. 2.	1. 2.
H.	(Identify a set of terms YOU think should be included) Term 1 *versus* Term 2	1. 2.	1. 2.
I.	(Identify a second set of terms YOU think should be included) Term 1 *versus* Term 2	1. 2.	1. 2.

4. Name four things you hope to learn about assessment from this workbook?

   I wish to learn _____

   I hope to learn _____

   I want to learn more about _____

   An important aspect of assessment I need to know more about in order to be a good diagnostician is _____

References

American Speech-Language-Hearing Association. (n.d.). *Assessment and evaluation of speech-language disorders in schools*. Retrieved May 14, 2018 from https://www.asha.org/SLP/Assessment-and-Evaluation-of-Speech-Language-Disorders-in-Schools/

Kratcoski, A. M. (1998). Guidelines for using portfolios in assessment and evaluation. *Language, Speech, and Hearing Services in Schools, 29*, 3–10.

Olswang, L. B., & Bain, B. A. (1994). Data collection: Monitoring children's treatment progress. *American Journal of Speech and Hearing Research, 3*(3), 53–64.

Westby, C. E., Stevens Dominguez, M., & Oetter, P. (1996). A performance/competence model of observational assessment. *Language, Speech, and Hearing Services in Schools, 27*, 144–156.

CHAPTER 2

Referrals

Who

Most all work settings will require a referral source for testing. On occasion and usually only if a site does not file insurance, a medical referral is not needed. As will be discussed more in the billing chapter (Chapter 13), medical referrals are needed for insurance filing purposes. Referrals also give the evaluator some information on the client prior to testing. If a client does not complete a case history form prior to the scheduled evaluation appointment, it is very difficult to determine what question(s) need to be answered during the evaluation. A referral can give the diagnostician some insight into the problem area(s). Referrals can be from a variety of professionals such as psychologists, physicians, school system employee, early interventionists, other service providers, or counselors, just to name a few. When a person recommends someone to see a speech-language pathologist (SLP) or audiologist, that is considered a referral. The medical definition of referral is "the process of directing or redirecting (as a medical case or a patient) to an appropriate specialist or agency for definitive treatment" (Referral [medical def. 1], n.d.). Based on that definition, a referral could be made by anyone, including family members and friends. A person may also make a connection with a practice on their own which is known as a self-referral. However, it is very common for someone to inquire about services and be told by the site that they will need to contact their primary care physician to have a referral sent in before they can be evaluated.

Clinicians often make referrals to other professionals. Following an evaluation, it is common for a clinician to determine that a client needs additional areas of assessment or follow-up; thus referring the client to another professional or entity. Any health care provider working in the United States will have a National Provider Identifier (NPI) number (Regulations and guidance, n.d). This number is used when filing insurance and you will likely see it on referral forms.

What

Referrals received by the SLP or audiologist provide more information about the potential patient. Typically, referrals include demographic information (name, date of birth, address, phone number) as well as the reason for the referral (e.g., speech delay, stroke, language disorders) and other diagnoses if applicable. Most often we think about referrals in

```
                        SAMPLE REFERRAL FORM
Referring Office/Physician Name: _____
Referring Office Address: _____
Referring Office Phone: _____ Referring Office Fax: _____

PLEASE INCLUDE ALL PATIENT DEMOGRAPHICS & INSURANCE INFORMATION

Patient Name: _____
D.O.B: _____ Guardian/Parents Name (if applicable): _____
Patient Address: _____
City/State: _____
Phone#: _____ Alternate#: _____
Insurance Company: _____
Policy/ID #: _____ Group#: _____
Insurance Tel#: _____
Reason for Referral:
_____ Hearing Evaluation
_____ Amplification
_____ Auditory Processing Disorder Evaluation (APD) Age 8–18
_____ Speech/Language Evaluation
_____ Speech Language Therapy
Brief description of problem:

Referring Physician's Signature:

NPI#:                          Print Physician Name:              Date:

Please fax this referral to (xxx) xxx-xxxx
```

Figure 2–1. Intake referral form. This form is a sample of a referral that you may receive to set up an evaluation.

the medical setting; however, referrals can be used in many settings to provide additional and important patient information. For example, a school SLP could use a referral form that is given to teachers to help identify students who need an evaluation (Prath, 2017). In the world of electronic health records (an electronic version of information on the patient), it is very common to receive visit notes for one or multiple visits from a physician's office visit. The more information that is provided on the referral, the more prepared a clinician can be for the evaluation. A sample incoming referral form is provided in Figure 2–1.

When clinicians observe or find something that they feel needs more follow-up, they may refer to other providers. For instance, if an SLP were to see a 4-year-old child who is having trouble grasping a large crayon to color, the SLP may refer the child to an occupational therapist (a therapist who works with a patient on activities of daily living: writing, fine-motor activities, using adaptive equipment for ease of daily living tasks) for further evaluation (About occupational therapy, n.d.). A sample outgoing referral is provided in Figure 2–2.

When referring to other providers or agencies, you must have the permission of the client (if over 18 years of age) or guardian (if under 18 years of age or mentally incapable of caring for themselves). The Health Insurance Portability and Accountability Act (HIPAA) gives specific guidelines on when and what information can be shared between referral

```
                           SAMPLE OUTGOING REFERRAL FORM
  Referring Office/Provider Name: _____
  Referring Office Address: _____
  Referring Office Phone: _____  Referring Office Fax: _____

  PLEASE INCLUDE ALL PATIENT DEMOGRAPHICS & INSURANCE INFORMATION

  Patient Name: _____
  D.O.B: _____ Guardian/Parents Name (if applicable): _____
  Patient Address: _____
  City/State: _____
  Phone#: _____ Alternate#: _____
  Insurance Company: _____
  Policy/ID #: _____Group#: _____
  Insurance Tel#: _____
  Reason for Referral:

  Referring Provider's Signature:

  NPI#:                           Print Provider Name:              Date:

  Please call with questions: (xxx) xxx-xxxx
```

Figure 2–2. Outgoing referral form. This form is a sample of a referral that you may make to an outside practitioner, provider, or agency.

agencies (Privacy and security information, 2016). There is potential for fines and even jail time if a professional does not adhere to the HIPAA guidelines. During the evaluation or at any time you would like to refer a client, you should discuss with the client or guardian what you are seeing and why you are interested in referring him/her. Sometimes a list of providers can be given to the client or guardian to contact his/her own without needing a referral; however, it is most often helpful to send a referral directly to the provider. When you send that information, you must have the client or guardian's written permission to share information about the client.

Why

Referrals can be both sent and received. We need referrals from physicians because insurance companies require the involvement of the client's medical team. Many insurances, such as Medicare and Blue Cross Blue Shield, require referrals from a physician for speech/language and/or audiology testing for the insurance company to pay for the visit (Ogden, 2017). Referrals also provide us with some background information in order to better prepare for the evaluation. As SLPs or audiologists, we specialize only in the field of communication; however, there are many other areas that clients may need additional information or assistance. Oftentimes, clients and family members are not aware of services that may be provided or needed and you as the clinician may be the first person that recognizes an area of need.

When

Referrals to you from other providers will ideally occur prior to scheduling a client, as referrals are often the first point in finding out information about an indivudal. In some instances, a client or individual may initiate an appointment and then get the referral; but from a billing standpoint, the referral should always be received prior to the initial appointment.

Referrals can occur at any time. Oftentimes, during an evaluation the clinician will note areas of additional concern; however, referrals can also happen as part of the therapy process.

Where

Referrals come from various outside agencies or even potential clients. Along those same lines, as a clinician, you may send referrals to different providers. Most often, referrals from speech-language pathology and audiology are sent to physicians, physical therapists, occupational therapists, school systems, counselors, and social workers. However, this list is very small in comparison to the vast array of places clients may be referred from.

How

Referrals should be in written format—even if that written format is sent through an electronic health record. This is because referrals may need to be reviewed at various times or even produced if audited by an insurance group. If a referral occurs only over, the phone there may not be a long-standing record of that referral. It is easiest to consistently use the same referral process (e.g., forms) so that other providers are familiar with your referral process and ensure you have all the needed information. In the same manner, when you use the same referral form to send information, providers will become more familiar with the information you send, which generally leads to fewer questions and/or missed information. Many offices have links on their websites that make it easier for outside sources to find needed information regarding the practice. If you are involved in the development of a referral form, we would encourage you to consider vital information you will need to receive as well as information that will be important to share with others should you not have the opportunity to speak with another provider directly. The sample referral forms in this chapter do not include the name of the business or contact information; however, forms should always prominently display this information.

Top 10 Terms

Referral

Referral source

National Provider Identifier (NPI)

Referral form
Demographic information
Occupational therapist
Reason for referral
Health Insurance Portability and Accountability Act (HIPAA)
Primary care physician
Electronic health records

Chapter Tips

1. Referrals are often needed for insurance/billing purposes. Referrals provide information from demographics (name, date of birth, address, phone number) to insurance information to areas of major concern.

2. Referrals can also include information you provide to the client/family and outside sources for additional evaluations/consultations. Often, a client will need another specialist or additional assistance from other service providers or entities. One of the easiest ways to provide that information is through the referral process. When sharing information about a client with another agency or professional, you must have the consent of the client or guardian. You should discuss the referral with the client/guardian and receive written permission to share information.

3. When you are sent a referral, you should utilize that information to help plan for the evaluation. Information such as date of birth can help you make sure you will be using the correct age group for standardized scores. Major area(s) of concern can help you start planning activities to elicit responses in order to determine if there is a communication delay, difference, or disorder.

Activities

2–1. Use the completed referral form to answer the following questions (Figure 2–3).
   1. How old is the client?
   2. What is the primary contact phone number?
   3. Who is referring the client?
   4. What is the physician's NPI number?
   5. What is the primary area of concern?
   6. Would you consider this more of a speech evaluation, language evaluation, or both?
   7. Does this referral cover an evaluation and subsequent treatment if needed?

WNC SHC, 2033 Uptown Rd., Anywhere, NC 42323, (555) 333-9847

Referring Office/Physician Name: _Dr. Clive Engelwood / Engelwood Pediatrics_

Referring Office Address: _____123 State Street_____

Referring Office Phone: __555-333-1234_____ Referring Office Fax: __555-333-1235

PLEASE INCLUDE ALL PATIENT DEMOGRAPHICS & INSURANCE INFORMATION

Patient Name: _____Radie Rice_____

D.O.B: _8-23-14_____ Guardian/Parents Name (if applicable): Will and Jill Rice_____

Patient Address: _____332 Oak St._____

City/State: _____Anywhere, NC 42323_____

Phone#: _____555-333-4848_____ Alternate#_____555-333-2448_

Insurance Company: _____BCBS_____

Policy/ID #: _____2469394x_____Group#: _____14349_____

Insurance Tel#: _____800-800-8001_____

Reason for Referral:

_____ Hearing Evaluation

_____ Amplification

_____ Auditory Processing Disorder Evaluation (APD) Age 8-18

__X___ Speech/Language Evaluation

__X___ Speech Language Therapy

Brief description of problem:

Has 10 words – only parents understand what he is saying.

Referring Physician's Signature: *Clive Englewood*

NPI#:   12387438   Print Physician Name: Clive Engelwood   Date: 7/16/11

Please fax this referral to (555) 333-9849

Figure 2–3. Completed sample intake referral form. This is an example of a completed intake referral form.

2–2. Read the following scenarios and match the service provider/entity you would refer to.

1. Primary care physician
2. Social worker
3. School
4. Physical therapist
5. Occupational therapist

_____ A. An elderly client cannot continue coming to therapy because he/she cannot afford gas to get to treatment.

_____ B. A child just failed a hearing evaluation and has a history of ear infections.

_____ C. A family just moved to the area and their preschooler is turning 3 in 4 months. The child needs speech/language services as well as occupational therapy.

_____ D. A client has arthritis and can no longer hold eating utensils.

_____ E. A client has been diagnosed with Parkinson's disease and is having problems walking.

Answers to Activities

2–1

1. 3 years, 1 month
2. 555–333–4848
3. Dr. Clive Englewood/Englewood Pediatrics
4. 12387438
5. Lack of words and clarity of speech
6. Language—only using 10 words; speech—only the child's parents can understand the child.
7. Yes, both evaluation and treatment are checked. If only evaluation was checked and it was determined the child qualified for services, then another referral would be needed to approve speech/language treatment.

2–2

A = 2. Social worker: social workers can assist people with locating resources to assist with various issues in their lives.

B = 1. Primary care physician: ultimately an ear, nose, and throat referral may be warranted; however, most insurances require a primary care physician referral to a specialist.

C = 3. School: school systems are required to serve children ages 3 to 21 when a client qualifies for services.

D = 5. Occupational therapist: occupational therapists assist with fine-motor issues.

E = 4. Physical therapist: physical therapists assist with gross-motor issues.

Wrap-Up

1. Two referral forms are provided here for you (Figures 2–4 and 2–5). Come up with a scenario you may encounter in the evaluation process and complete both the intake referral form (what information were you provided with prior to the evaluation) and the outgoing referral form (what information would you give to the service provider to whom you are referring).

   What information were you provided that helped you get ready for the evaluation?

   _____

   _____

   _____

   _____

REFERRAL FORM

Referring Office/Physician Name: _____
Referring Office Address: _____
Referring Office Phone: _____ Referring Office Fax: _____

PLEASE INCLUDE ALL PATIENT DEMOGRAPHICS & INSURANCE INFORMATION

Patient Name: _____
D.O.B: _____ Guardian/Parents Name (if applicable): _____
Patient Address: _____
City/State: _____
Phone#: _____ Alternate#: _____
Insurance Company: _____
Policy/ID #: _____ Group#: _____
Insurance Tel#: _____
Reason for Referral:
____Hearing Evaluation
____Amplification
____Auditory Processing Disorder Evaluation (APD) Age 8–18
____Speech/Language Evaluation
____Speech Language Therapy
Brief description of problem:

Referring Physician's Signature:

NPI#: _____ Print Physician Name _____ Date: _____

Please fax this referral to (xxx) xxx-xxxx

Figure 2–4. Intake referral form. Complete the form with the information you were provided prior to the evaluation.

OUTGOING REFERRAL FORM

Referring Office/Provider Name: _____
Referring Office Address: _____
Referring Office Phone: _____ Referring Office Fax: _____

PLEASE INCLUDE ALL PATIENT DEMOGRAPHICS & INSURANCE INFORMATION

Patient Name: _____
D.O.B: _____ Guardian/Parents Name (if applicable): _____
Patient Address: _____
City/State: _____
Phone#: _____ Alternate#: _____
Insurance Company: _____
Policy/ID #: _____ Group#: _____
Insurance Tel#: _____
Reason for Referral:

Referring Provider's Signature:

NPI#:   Print Provider Name: Date:

Please call with questions: (xxx) xxx-xxxx

Figure 2–5. Outgoing referral form. Complete the form with the information would you give to the service provider to whom you are referring.

What information should you give to the client/guardian?

_____

_____

_____

_____

What information did you share with the service provider to whom you are referring?

_____

_____

_____

_____

References

About occupational therapy. (n.d.). Retrieved February 20, 2018, from https://www.aota.org/About-Occupational-Therapy.aspx

Ogden, K. (2017). Coding and billing 101. *The ASHA Leader, 10*, 34–36.

Prath, S. (2017). Make the speech referral process work for you. *The ASHA Leader, 10*, 38–39.

Privacy and security information. (2016, June 21). Retrieved September 12, 2017, from https://www.cms.gov/Regulations-and-Guidance/Administrative-Simplification/HIPAA-ACA/PrivacyandSecurityInformation.html

Referral [medical def. 1]. (n.d.). In *Merriam-Webster.com*. Retrieved July 03, 2017, from https://www.merriam-webster.com/dictionary/referral

Regulations and guidance. (n.d.). Retrieved October 1, 2017, from https://www.cms.gov/Regulations-and-Guidance/Administrative-Simplification/NationalProvIdentStand/downloads/NPIfinalrule.pdf

CHAPTER 3

Intake and Interview

Who

All initial assessments begin with a review of the intake material completed by the family or client prior to the assessment appointment. The information on past and current functioning level provided on an intake or case history form is used in the planning of the specific assessment. Intake material will vary somewhat depending on the age of the individual being assessed or the specific needs of the site. An intake form for a young child will likely include identifying information, concerns prompting the assessment, prenatal history, birth history, developmental history, medical history, and communication/social history. The intake form for a school-aged child would be similar to that for a young child with the addition of an educational history component. An adult intake form would include the identifying information, concerns prompting the assessment, medical history, work history, and perhaps health habits (such as use of tobacco, caffeine, alcohol/drug, and amount of exercise and diet). Intake forms vary in the amount of information requested and the organization of the form. This is probably not something you will personally develop, but rather something you will utilize from your work site. Using the headings of the intake form can facilitate the organization of your interview.

In the initial interview of the family member or client by the clinician, the material provided on the intake form is verified, clarified, and expanded. After introducing himself/herself, the clinician will make sure the address, contact phone number, name, age, referral source, and so forth are accurate. Any questions raised by the intake responses will be addressed and follow-up questions or concerns will be raised. The clinician should take care not to verbally ask all the questions from the intake form, but rather to use the interview to supplement what has already been provided on the intake form. The family and client should also be given ample opportunity to ask questions and raise topics in the interview. The time required for an interview can vary. Mar and Sall (1999) suggest spending at least 30 min when conducting an interview with clients who have multiple disabilities, including those with severe or profound intellectual impairments and deafblindness.

The intake form and interview are the first time the client, family, and clinician will begin to develop a therapeutic relationship. In formulating a theoretical framework to describe the ideal attitude and characteristics of a speech-language pathologist based on interviews of adult clients, Fourie (2009) identified the therapeutic qualities of being understanding, being gracious, being erudite (being knowledgeable and being able to communicate that knowledge), and being inspiring as well as the therapeutic actions of being confident, being soothing, being practical, and being empowering. The clinician should be cognizant of the importance of the professional impression he/she is making.

What

As the intake form is provided by the site, the remainder of the chapter will focus on the interview process. Typically, an interview will begin by making sure the paperwork is in order. The consent to evaluate needs to be explained and signed, the client/family needs to have received written notice of their rights, and site-specific consent for things, such as audio or video recording, needs to be obtained.

Next, the identifying information from the intake form is verified. The reason for the referral, usually a part of the intake information, is discussed. The clinician might say, "Tell me what concerns brought you here today?" or "What do you hope will be the outcome of this evaluation session?" The questions generated from the reason for seeking the evaluation should drive and focus the assessment. Ultimately, when the diagnostic session is completed, the client/family will be provided with information to address their concerns. This might also be the time when the clinician clarifies the scope of what a speech/language assessment will and will not be able to address. It is important that expectations of the client/family correspond to information the clinician is able to obtain.

Following the order of the intake form, the various pertinent histories (e.g., prenatal, birth, developmental, medical, communication/social, educational, work, and/or health habits) are clarified and expanded in sequence. The amount of time spent on each specific history section will vary depending on the particular individual. Generally, a good amount of time is devoted to the communication history. Questions a clinician might ask himself/herself as he/she progresses through each history section are as follows:

1. Were there difficulties during the pregnancy or birth; and if yes, can I describe these difficulties and their effects?
2. Were development milestones met at appropriate ages; and if no, were the delays broad based or restricted to a specific kind of development (e.g., fine motor, gross motor, speech, or language)?
3. Have there been or do there continue to be medical concerns; and can I describe the depth and breadth of these medical issues?
4. Are there factors that have resulted in the current communication strengths and limitations?
5. Who/what are/is the client's preferred partners, preferred modes of communication, ability to communicate with peers, play level, needs for communication, and typical settings for communication?
6. What educational strengths, supports, and needs have shaped and continue to impact the individual's communication?

7. What work related strengths, supports, and needs have shaped and continue to shape the individual's communication?
8. How are past or current health habits affected and how do they continue to influence the client's communication?

At the closing of the interview, the clinician provides a brief description of the procedures that will occur in the evaluation, asks if there is any additional information the informant wishes to share, and asks if there are questions that can be answered before the evaluation begins. Asking if there is anything they wish to add allows the family the freedom to take the interview in a new direction. An example of this would be a mother remembering to mention how her son had been evaluated the week before at a local hospital and she was wondering if the results would be the same.

Why

The interview sets the stage and provides important information for the rest of the assessment. It reminds us that the strengths and weaknesses seen today have been influenced by events of the past. It also reminds us that a communication disorder affects not just a single individual but the entire family. It reminds us that communication is not an isolated skill but is vital to the person's entire life. It also reminds us as clinicians to be holistic in our assessment.

When

The initial interview has been the focus of this chapter. It occurs prior to the initial evaluation and focuses on history as well as current level of functioning. Additional interviews can and should occur at any time throughout the therapy process. These would focus more on current and future impact of therapy. Similar behaviors can be employed in any interview. These facilitating behaviors will be addressed in the How section.

Where

The interview needs to be conducted in a quiet and confidential area. You are asking the individual to provide personal and confidential information. At times, the telling of this information is painful to recount even after many years. The clinician should be aware of where the informant is in the stages of grief as this can affect the information provided. These stages include denial, guilt, depression, anger, bargaining, and acceptance (Mandell & Fiscus, 1981). An individual's progress through the stages varies, including time at each stage, order of the stages, stages that are never experienced, and stages that are experienced repeatedly.

The most common places to hold an interview are a therapy room, a client's home, or a client's hospital/rehabilitation residence room. Always guard against holding interviews in inappropriate places, such as hallways, waiting rooms, bathrooms, busy classrooms, and lunch tables.

How

There is no easy answer to how to do an effective interview as it is a multidimensional and individualistic process. The clinician should strive to be prepared, to be organized, to be culturally sensitive, and to be present. The interviewer is serving multiple roles including: (1) encouraging the informant's participation and guiding the informant through the process; (2) seeking, verifying, and integrating information; and (3) sharing information and addressing questions raised by the informant.

Clinician behaviors can facilitate or impede an interview. Table 3–1 provides a listing of clinician behaviors that aid the interview process as well as examples and nonexamples of each behavior.

Table 3–1. Clinician Behaviors That Aid the Interview Process

Facilitating Clinician Interview Behaviors	Examples—Things You Should Do	Nonexamples—Things You Should Avoid
Active listening	Focusing on the speaker, nodding, maintaining eye contact, and saying "mmm hmm" to signify you are listening.	Looking away every time someone goes by, focusing on your list of questions, and interrupting or finishing sentences for others.
Positive affect	Smiling, nodding, and maintaining eye contact.	Frowning, checking your watch repeatedly, yawning, and slouching in your chair.
Open-ended question	"What is a typical day for him?"	Using many closed questions such as, "Does he go to school? Where?"
Follow-up question	"Who else besides yourself understands him well?	"More?"
Nonleading question	"What changes have you observed in her speech since the stroke?"	"She has made few improvements since the stroke, right?"
Summarizing	"You noted that he has difficulty in school with English and social studies, but is preforming above grade level in science and math."	"OK I got it, let's move on."
Paraphrasing	"I heard you say that his disfluencies increase during holidays or times when he is very tired."	"I wrote down that you said, 'Tom gets stuck on his words when he is up too late three days in a row.'"
Asking for confirmation	"The medicine he is currently taking is _____. Is that correct?"	"He is on medication—that's all I need to know."

continues

Table 3–1. (continued)

Facilitating Clinician Interview Behaviors	Examples—Things You Should Do	Nonexamples—Things You Should Avoid
Good communication skills	Using good grammar, speaking at an appropriate loudness, and maintaining appropriate personal space with the informant	Using space fillers such as "uh," "um," or "you know,"; "me and my supervisor found the same thing"; and playing with your hair while you interview.
Redirecting	"That was a good example of the behavior; now can you share. . ."	"That was not what I asked you—you need to tell me about his current behavior."
Integrating information	"Looking at all the developmental ages you provided, it appears that speech was the only area of development delay."	"You said he walked at 16 months and said his first word at 24 months."

Top 10 Terms

Birth history
Communication/social history
Developmental history
Facilitating clinician interview behaviors
Health habits
Intake form
Interview
Medical history
Prenatal history
Stages of grief

Chapter Tips

1. The more you know and understand about the culture of the individual and family prior to the interview, the more successful your interview process will likely be. A resource that can be helpful is *Culture and Clinical Care* (Lipson & Dibble, 2005). This book provides information concerning health beliefs and practices (including verbal and nonverbal communication) for 35 cultures.

2. Be prepared with questions you think will be appropriate, but do not use these questions as a script. You need to follow the flow of the interview and not be wed to your prepared question list.

3. If someone gives information you do not know about or understand, ask them to clarify and explain. For example, if the individual has used a drug you are not familiar with, ask about it and then research the material to be sure you are providing accurate information in the report.

Activities

3–1. The interview is the time the clinician makes his/her first impression. Listed in Table 3–2 are several positive characteristics of a clinician. Next to each characteristic identify two or three things a clinician might say or do in an initial interview that would reflect each characteristic.

Table 3–2. Positive Characteristics of a Clinician

Characteristic	What a Clinician Could Say or Do to Reflect the Characteristic
Professional	
Active listener	
Caring	
Organized	
Unbiased	
Culturally sensitive	
Knowledgeable	
Ethical	

3–2. An intake form for a young child will often ask parents to identify the age when the child exhibited certain developmental milestones. A clinician should never provide the family with anything they have not read and understood. Use a reliable source (e.g., your developmental textbooks or ASHA's website) to give approximate age of acquisition for the milestones in Table 3–3. For an interesting examination of a stage model approach to speech/language development, read the Prutting (1979) article. Then in Table 3–3, identify three additional milestones you believe are important to ask about and document.

Table 3–3. Typical Age of Developmental Milestones

Milestone	Typical Age of Acquisition
Babbled	
Used single words	
Combined two words	
Pointed at pictures in book	
Crawled	
Walked	
Toilet trained	
Responded to name	
Drank from a cup	
Cooed	

Answers to Activity

3–1

Table 3–4. Answers to Activity 3–1

Characteristic	What a Clinician Could Say or Do to Reflect the Characteristic
Professional	Clean and appropriate dress. Firm handshake. Good model of communication including pragmatics, grammar, articulation, loudness, and so forth.
Active listener	Maintains eye contact. Asks appropriate follow-up questions. Restates and asks for confirmation.
Caring	Interested in the whole client. Is empathetic (versus sympathetic). Explains what will happen during the assessment. Asks and values the client's responses. Has tissues available.
Organized	Has all materials and equipment ready for use. Starts and ends on time. Asks for information in a logical sequence.
Unbiased	Asks open-ended questions. Withholds judgement. Phrases questions as to not influence the answer ("How does John interact with his sister?" vs. "His sister talks for John, doesn't she?").

continues

Table 3–4. (*continued*)

Characteristic	What a Clinician Could Say or Do to Reflect the Characteristic
Culturally sensitive	Ask the parent/caregiver how they wish to be addressed. Allows sufficient time for response, because wait time before answering questions differs across cultures.
Knowledgeable	Explains what is going to occur in the evaluation. Knows the name and purpose of assessment measures that will be used. Answers client/family questions in a clear manner.
Ethical	Provides a confidential space to hold the interview. Explains the consent to evaluate forms. Practices within a speech-language pathologist's scope of practice.

3–2

Table 3–5. Answers to Activity 3–2

Milestone	Typical Age of Acquisition
Babbled	4–7 months
Used single words	12 months
Combined two words	24 months
Pointed at pictures in book	19–24 months
Crawled	7–12 months
Walked	13–18 months
Toilet trained	18 months–3 years (culturally dependent)
Responded to name	7–12 months
Drank from a cup	7–12 months
Cooed	Birth–3 months

Wrap-Up

1. As a clinician, you need to be aware of your own health beliefs and practices, especially those concerning communication. The five areas identified in bold were selected from the many topics presented in the Lipson and Dibble (2005) text. Write a few sentences describing the unwritten "rules" **your** culture practices for each of the following topics. Identify how another culture views the "rules" differently.

Personal Space
Your culture's view:
_____
_____
_____

Another culture's view:
_____
_____
_____

Touch
Your culture's view:
_____
_____
_____

Another culture's view:
_____
_____
_____

Time orientation
Your culture's view:
_____
_____
_____

Another culture's view:
_____
_____
_____

Eye contact

Your culture's view:

_____
_____
_____

Another culture's view:

_____
_____
_____

Gestures

Your culture's view:

_____
_____
_____

Another culture's view:

_____
_____
_____

2. It can be difficult to ask information in a professional manner. The following are four poorly worded interview questions. How would you ask for this information in a professional manner?

"Does your child sit in front of a television screen all day?"

_____
_____

"Is there a man you're not married to living with you and your children?"

_____
_____

"Why did you wait so long before you brought him in to be evaluated?"

_____
_____

"Why are you giving the individual water to drink when it says in his file that he aspirates when given liquids?"

_____

_____

3. A family member will sometimes ask hard questions during an interview. Write a response to the following four questions asked by a family member in an interview.

"Did I cause this? Is it my fault?"

_____

_____

_____

_____

"How long until my nonverbal child will talk?"

_____

_____

_____

_____

"Will my husband have to stay on this restricted diet the rest of his life?"

_____

_____

_____

_____

"How come the doctor didn't identify the problem sooner?"

_____

_____

_____

_____

"What's wrong with my child?"

References

Fourie, R. J. (2009). Qualitative study of the therapeutic relationship in speech and language therapy: Perspectives of adults with acquired communication and swallowing disorders. *International Journal of Language Communication Disorders, 44*(6), 979–999.

Lipson, J. G., & Dibble, S. L. (Eds.). (2005). *Culture & clinical care*. San Francisco, CA: UCSF Nursing Press.

Mandell, C. J., & Fiscus, E. (1981). *Understanding exceptional people*. St. Paul, MN: West Group.

Mar, H. H., & Sall, N. (1999). *Dimensions of communication*. New York, NY: Saint Luke's/Roosevelt Hospital Center, Developmental Disabilities Center (ED444291).

Prutting, C. A. (1979). Process/pra/,ses/n: The action of moving forward progressively from one point to another on the way to completion. *Journal of Speech and Hearing Disorders, 44*(1), 3–30.

CHAPTER 4

Oral-Facial Examinations

Who

The oral-facial examination is important for any client referred for a communication disorder evaluation (Johnson-Root, 2015). We need to determine if the oral structures are intact and functioning at an appropriate level for speech purposes. No matter who you are assessing with an oral-facial examination, you need to embrace the philosophy of universal precautions by being committed to appropriate infection control practices (Centers for Disease Control, 2007). Universal precautions involve treating every client as though he/she is infectious. Infection control practices most relevant to assessment include washing hands, using new tongue depressors, disinfecting/sterilizing equipment and spaces, and wearing personal protective equipment such as gloves when you are going to come in physical contact with the mouth or any bodily fluids. All these precautions are taken to decrease the likelihood of spreading pathogens. Employing these precautions is critical for the protection of clients and clinicians alike.

What

There are a number of terms used to describe the examination of the structure and function of the oral mechanism. The terms include oral-facial examination, oroperipheral examination, oral peripheral examination, oral mechanism examination, and oral exam. Oral peripheral examination is defined as:

> Inspection of the mouth to determine its structural and functional adequacy for speech. It includes: (a) lips: size, symmetry, mobility, and possible presence of scars; (b) jaws: symmetry, position at rest, and rate of movement; (c) teeth: occlusion while at rest and general condition; (d) tongue: size relative to the rest of the mouth, swallowing patterns, symmetry while at rest and in motion, and mobility and rate of mobility for protrusion, retraction, elevation, depression, and lateral movements; (e) hard palate: shape, width, height, and possible scarring; (f) soft palate: closure; size, symmetry, movement up and back, and laterally, and possible scarring; and (g) fauces: status of tonsils, width of isthmus, scarring and general condition of the oropharynx. (Nicolosi, Harryman, & Kresheck, 1978, pp. 145–146)

The examination of the structures includes: (1) overall facial appearance, (2) lips, (3) teeth, (4) tongue, (5) hard palate, (6) velum (soft palate), and (7) tonsils. In general, we are looking for symmetry, condition, size, and color of each structure (for an in-depth examination of the oral-facial examination, see Johnson-Root, 2015). If any of these factors are not judged to be within normal limits, then an indication of the difference is recorded. Table 4–1 provides a set of questions to consider for each structure.

In evaluating the function of pertinent structures, the clinician instructs the client to perform specified movements or sounds and records whether the movements or sounds are judged to be within normal limits. Telling the client to move his/her structures or to produce specified sounds may be augmented by demonstrating the movements or sounds. In general, movement, precision, strength, and degree of effort are evaluated for relevant structure. In addition to examining the function of specific structures, swallowing behavior and rapid overlapping movements that involve multiple structures are also examined. Table 4–2 provides examples of functions assessed by structure.

Table 4–1. Questions to Consider When Evaluating Certain Oral Structures

Structure	Symmetry, Condition, Size, and Color
Overall facial appearance	Is the right and left side of the face symmetrical? Are there scars? Are there tremors or ticks? Are the features normal in size or proximity to other features? Is the face flushed or abnormally pale?
Lips	Are the lips symmetrical? Do the lips meet? Is there drooping of one side at rest? Is there drooling? Is the length normal? Are there scars?
Teeth	Is the occlusion normal (vs. underbite or overbite)? Are teeth in good condition? Are teeth missing, rotated, or jumbled? Does client wear dentures or braces?
Tongue	Is the frenulum excessively short? Is the tongue symmetrical? Is thickness within normal limits? Is color appropriate?
Hard palate	Is palate symmetrical? Are height and contour too flat or too pointed and narrow? Is there a cleft or repaired cleft? Is palate discolored?
Velum (soft palate) Tonsils	Is uvula absent, bifurcated (split in two), or deviated to one side? Are the tonsils present? Are they inflamed and/or excessively large?

Table 4–2. Examples of Functions Assessed for Each Oral Structure

Structure	Function: Movement, Precision, Strength, Degree of Effort
Overall facial appearance	Not Applicable.
Lips	Can lips be protruded? Can lips be retracted to the left, right, and bilaterally? Can client rapidly produce repetition of /pʌ/?
Teeth	Not Applicable.
Tongue	Can client stick tongue out and retract? When sticking out, is tongue pulled in the middle (by the attachment to the frenulum)? When sticking tongue out, are tremors observed? Can he/she move tongue side to side? Up and down? Is movement slow or restricted? When pushing against a tongue depressor at each side and up and down, does it demonstrate appropriate strength? Can client rapidly produce repetitions of /tʌ/?
Hard palate	Not Applicable.
Velum (soft palate)	Is the velum moving during the repetition and prolongation of an /ɑ/?
Tonsils	Not Applicable.
Swallowing behavior	Given a sip of water and holding the lips parted, does water get pushed forward during the swallow (indicating a tongue thrust)?
Rapid overlapping movements	Can client produce rapid repetition of /pʌtəkə/ (after demonstration by clinician) without errors, halting, or slow production?

There are numerous forms available for recording your examination of the structure and function of the oral structures (see Hegde, 2008, pp. 344–351, or Shipley & McAfee, 2016, pp. 145–148, for samples of oral-facial examination forms). Typically, a structure is identified and then, in the same space, the integrity of the structure and its ability to function appropriately are recorded. While structure and function are evaluated at one time and often recorded in one place on a recording form, it is possible to have an intact structure and weak functioning or inadequate structure and strong functioning. Thus, you need to evaluate structure and function independently. Your work site will most likely have a form available for recording the oral-facial examination information.

Integrated within an oral-facial examination is the evaluation of the diadochokinetic rate (DDK). The DDK looks at rapid movement of the lips (by repetition of /pʌ/), the tongue (by repetition of /tʌ/), the velum (by repetition of /kʌ/), and the coordination of these varied movements (by repetition of /pʌtəkə/). DDK can be measured in several ways. Fletcher (1972) provided norms for the number of seconds it took children ages 6 to 13 years to produce 20 repetitions of /pʌ/, /tʌ/, and /kʌ/ as well as 10 repetitions of /pʌtəkə/. Using the data in the article, the clinician can compare the client's number of repetitions to the means and standard deviations of the normed sample. It is more common for clinicians to make a gross judgment of the client's ability to produce the rapid speech movements. Clinicians may ask clients to produce the movements from between 5 to 20 times while timing them on a stopwatch and counting the number of repetitions completed. The clinician then makes a judgment as to whether the rate appeared normal or slow.

Why

The reason for doing an oral-facial examination is to determine the structural integrity and the ability of the structures to function in a manner necessary for speech production/swallowing. The results of the oral-facial examination have an impact on the other procedures completed in the evaluation as well as the interpretation of results, recommendations, and referrals.

When

While an oral-facial examination can be done at any time, it is usually completed in the initial assessment. Again, there are no hard and fast rules about when it is conducted during the initial assessment. Many clinicians perform the oral-facial examination toward the beginning of the session.

The information gathered from this procedure can help the clinician focus on certain aspects during the remainder of the evaluation. Knowing a child demonstrates groping while performing voluntary movements of the lips and tongue will alert the clinician to aspects of articulation (a consideration of apraxia) on which to focus. Knowing a client has drooling at rest will alert the clinician to potential swallowing issues. Knowing a client has an overbite and tongue thrust will alert the clinician to a potential /θ/ and /ð/ substitution for /s/ and /z/.

The need for a referral can result from an oral-facial examination. An excessively short frenulum that does not allow for adequate production of /l/ could lead to a referral to a pediatrician for further assessment. A white line on the top of the hard palate when a light is shown on it along with a lack of solid structure behind the palate when gently probed by the clinician and excessive nasality would prompt a referral to the doctor to determine if a submucus cleft is present. The results of the oral-facial examination must be integrated into the other aspects of the assessment and be a part of the comprehensive oral and written reports.

Where

This is one procedure that is commonly performed in a segregated treatment room or in the client's hospital room. The need for infection control procedures makes it desirable to have a more controlled environment.

How

First and foremost, always follow infection control practices. Positioning is important in an oral-facial examination. The client's oral structures are best viewed while the client is sitting upright with good posture. The clinician should be at the client's level (rather than above and looking down at the structures) and move off his/her chair and/or have the client tilt his/her head to help the oral structures be viewed more clearly. The tongue depressor is used to gently hold the tongue down out of the way for viewing the velum during phonation and for gauging strength of the tongue. Light from a small flash light helps illuminate the oral cavity. The clinician should explain what the client is to do, why he/she is being instructed to do the tasks, and provide demonstration when appropriate. The procedures may be modified depending on the age and language abilities of the client. For example, a more gamelike approach of face making in the mirror may be used with young children. Also "buttercup-buttercup-buttercup" can be used to assess rapid movements for young children's diadochokinetic rate instead of the preferred /pʌtəkə_pʌtəkə_pʌtəkə/. Demonstration of the movements or sounds can be appropriate for any age.

The following is a list of items you might want to have available:

- Case history form
- Consent form
- Disposable gloves (wear glove on your nondominant hand while your pen is in your dominant hand)
- Stopwatch (for DDK rate)
- Small flashlight
- Tongue depressor(s)
- Oral-facial exam recording form
- Pen and clipboard
- Hand sanitizer/sanitizing wipes
- Eye/mouth protection if you suspect that bodily fluids may spray or splash
- Gown/shoe coverings if you expect any contact with bodily fluids

Top 10 Terms

Diadochokinetic rate

Hard palate

Infection control

Lips

Oral-facial examination

Overall facial appearance

Teeth

Tongue

Universal precautions

Velum

Chapter Tips

1. Universal precautions are always essential to maintain during an oral exam. Properly disinfecting/cleaning your space and materials before and after an oral exam is critical (CDC, 2007). Remember to wash your hands before and after putting on gloves. When you remove gloves, keep the exposed surface turned inward. These precautions are important to protect your client, your family, and yourself.

2. I find it better to "tell" or "show" the client what I want them to do in an oral exam instead of "asking." "Pucker your lips" or "Show me how you would kiss mom" could be used instead of "Can you pucker your lips?" Telling seems to eliminate some of the "no" responses produced when directions are asked in question form.

3. As a student clinician or beginning clinician you need to develop a sense of what a "normal" oral cavity should look and function like. Take every opportunity to look in a variety of oral cavities and observe their functioning.

Activities

4–1. Answer the following questions based on this scenario. Ben, a 5-year-old male being seen in clinic for an articulation evaluation, spit saliva on the clinician as he made his sound. She had on gloves and calmly took a sanitizing wipe from her bag, wiped it off her arm, threw the wipe away, and continued with the assessment.

- Did the clinician do the right thing?

_____

_____

_____

_____

- Would you call her action universal precaution or infection control? Explain.

_____

_____

_____

_____

- Mom was watching the session and became annoyed stating, "Does she think my kid has a terrible disease he's going to give her?" What would you say to mom?

_____

_____

_____

_____

4–2. Develop your own Dos and Don'ts chart in Table 4–3. In column 1, list things you should do when conducting an oral-facial examination; and in column 2, list things you should not do. Compare your list to the one provided in the Answers to Activities section.

Table 4–3. Dos and Don'ts Chart

Dos	Don'ts

4–3. Explain to a family member where an identified anatomical structure lies in relations to another anatomical structure. Use Table 4–4 to record your responses.

Table 4–4. Chart Explaining Where an Identified Anatomical Structure Lies in Relationship to Another Anatomical Structure

Anatomical Structure	Relationship to Another Anatomical Structure Using Family-Friendly Terminology
Alveolar ridge	
Velopharyngeal port	
Vocal folds	
Velum	
Tonsils	
Nasal cavity	
Frenulum	
Uvula	

4–4. Think back to your phonetics class, why do we transcribe DDK as /pʌtəkə/ and not /pʌtʌkʌ/?

Answers to Activities

4–1.

The clinician's actions were appropriate. She followed the philosophy of universal precaution by practicing infection control. I would tell mom that universal precautions dictate that we treat saliva as potentially carrying disease. We do this universally with all clients as we do not know if an individual has a virus or other communicable disease. We clean up saliva as well as disinfect equipment and surfaces before and after every client and wear gloves when appropriate. We do this for the protection of the client as well as the protection of ourselves. We use these safety practices with all clients at all times.

4–2.

Table 4–5. Completed Answer Chart for the Do and Don't of an Oral Peripheral Exam

Do	Don't
Practice the procedures before you conduct the exam.	Giggle through the exam—practice enough so you are not self-conscious about doing an oral exam.

continues

Table 4–5. (*continued*)

Do	Don't
Gather your materials including gloves, tongue depressor, recording sheet, and flashlight (you might want to put together a kit of all needed materials for an oral exam).	Use single-use equipment more than once.
Disinfect and sterilize equipment before and after an oral exam.	Put your pen, flashlight, or fingers (or anything else) in your mouth.
Wear glove(s) and keep them sanitary.	Be gentle, but do not be afraid to use the tongue depressor to hold the tongue down or to the side.
Tell your client what will happen and why you are doing a procedure. Talk during the procedure.	Be afraid to move off your chair or reposition the clients mouth so you can better see.
Use age-appropriate language.	Be afraid to praise the client for participation or movement (unlike a norm based test).
Record information as you go.	Position the client lying down whenever possible.
Be careful when you remove your glove(s) to not touch the surface and keep the exposed side inward.	

4–3.

Table 4–6. Chart with Answers Explaining Where an Identified Anatomical Structure Lies in Relationship to Another Anatomical Structure

Anatomical structure	Relationship to Another Anatomical Structure Using Family-Friendly Terminology
Alveolar ridge	Directly behind the teeth (upper and lower) that hold the teeth sockets.
Velopharyngeal port	Opening between the oral cavity and nasal cavity in the back of the throat.
Vocal folds	Bands of tissue housed within the larynx or voice box behind the Adam's apple.
Velum	Also called the soft palate. The back of the roof of the mouth.

Table 4–6. (*continued*)

Anatomical structure	Relationship to Another Anatomical Structure Using Family-Friendly Terminology
Tonsils	In the back of the throat at both sides.
Nasal cavity	Area within the nose.
Frenulum	Tissue connecting floor of the mouth to the underside of the tongue.
Uvula	Tissue that hangs down in the back of the throat and vibrates when saying "ah."

4–4.

Remember back to your phonetics class that /ə/ is used in stress syllable, while /ɪ/ is used for unstressed syllable. Thus, the correct transcription is /pətəkə/ and not /pətəkə/.

Wrap-Up

1. Which term for the examination of the oral structures makes the most sense to you? Justify your selection.

    _____
    _____
    _____
    _____

2. These days, we all use the light from our cell phone when we need a flashlight. Why is it not a good idea to use your cell phone light to look into a client's mouth during an oral-facial exam? Is it appropriate to use the stop watch on your phone for timing the diadochokinetic rate?

    _____
    _____
    _____
    _____

3. Way back in 1995, Grube and Nunley surveyed 5,000 speech-language pathologists concerning their use of universal precautions during diagnostic

evaluations. Some of the questions and results from page 17 of their study are as follow.

- I wash my hands immediately before conducting the oral exam (54% always; 11% never).
- I wear gloves for the oral exam (43% always; 31% never).
- I wash my hands after removing gloves (60% always; 24% never).
- After the oral exam, are equipment/materials disinfected? (47% always; 30% never).

Ask three current speech-language clinicians or audiologists (in person or through email) to take these questions and tell you their thinking about universal precautions/infection control. Summarize the results from your three sources and discuss what you believe about universal precautions.

_____

_____

_____

_____

4. Sign your name here as a pledge to practice universal precautions.

_____

References

Centers for Disease Control. (2007). Guidelines for isolation precautions: Preventing transmission of infectious agents in healthcare settings 2007. Retrieved May 17, 2018, from https://www.cdc.gov/infectioncontrol/guidelines/index.html

Fletcher, S. G. (1972). Time-by-count measurement of diadochokinetic syllable rate. *Journal of Speech, Language, and Hearing Research, 15*, 736–770.

Grube, M. M., & Nunley, R. L. (1995). Current infection control practices in speech-language pathology. *American Journal of Speech-Language Pathology, 4*, 14–23.

Hegde, M. N. (2008). *Hegde's pocketguide to assessment in speech-language pathology* (3rd ed.). Clifton Park, NY: Delmar Learning.

Johnson-Root, A. A. (2015). *Oral-facial evaluation for speech-language pathology.* San Diego, CA: Plural.

Nicolosi, L., Harryman, E., & Kresheck, N. (1978). *Terminology of communication Disorders.* Baltimore, MD: Williams & Wilkins.

Shipley, K. G., & McAfee, J. G. (2016). *Assessment in speech-language pathology* (5th ed.). Boston, MA: Cengage Learning.

CHAPTER 5

Standardized Testing

Who

The focus of this chapter is the clinician as a selector, administrator, analyzer, and reporter of standardized test information. This is a critical component of being a competent diagnostician. Fulcher-Rood, Castilla-Earls, and Higginbotham (2018) found school-based clinicians utilized both standardized testing and informal testing during diagnostic assessment. However, they reported that standardized test results were more common in determining eligibility and severity.

What

The first step in the sequence is selecting an appropriate standardized test to administer. Start with what question(s) you wish to answer by using the test. Standardized tests can be used to address the following questions:

How does this client stand relative to similarly aged peers?

Are you looking for a broadly focused measure covering many areas of the suspected problem or a specifically targeted measure focusing on one specific aspect of the problem?

Does he/she qualify for services?

What is the severity level?

Next, select a reputable client-appropriate test. Reviewing all the psychometric characteristics of a standardized test are beyond the scope of this chapter (see Hegde & Pomaville, 2013, for a description of standardized test construction). In general, a reputable test is theoretically sound, valid (measures what it says it measures), reliable (measures consistently), and current (new or the most updated version). The test manual will be your source of this psychometric information (McCauley & Swisher, 1984). Practically speaking, you will select a reputable test from those available to you at your job site or within your organizational agency. A client-appropriate test is one whose norm groups represent a similar age and background of the client you are assessing. You usually use a standardized test because it allows you to compare the client's results to a sample of peers. The standardized test is always only one component of your assessment. Along with standardized testing, the use of measures including observation, structured tasks, dynamic assessment, and the analysis of conversational interactions provides relevant information for the clinician to develop a well-supported clinical interpretation (Plante, 1996). If no appropriate standardized tests are available, the informal evaluation tools noted above can allow you to make an informed clinical decision.

Step three is administering the test. The test manual is once again your primary source of information. Always read the instructions in the manual, gather any materials you need (including the test response recording form and test item booklet), and practice giving the test before you administer it to any client. Some tests will allow you to give an item more than once or provide additional information, while others do not. The manual will provide this kind of information, which is critical to administering the test in the standard manner that is the same for every test taker.

A few items of note about administering a standardized test include administering a practice item versus a scored test item, determining the client's age, the use of basal and ceiling items, and understanding a raw score.

A practice item and a testing item serve very different purposes in a standardized test. A practice item is used to demonstrate the task the client will be doing. It allows for the clinician to give feedback. It is generally an easy item so the clinician knows the client understands and can do the task he is being asked to do on the test items to come. The practice item(s) are not part of the client's score. On the other hand, the test items are presented exactly as specified in the manual, are scored and recorded on the test record form, and are given with no feedback regarding correctness.

As mentioned earlier, we use a standardized test to compare the client's score to a same-aged norm group. An accurate age in years and months is essential to giving and scoring the test. To figure age, start by recording the date you are administering the test in the order of year, month (January as 01 to December as 12), and day (the 1st as 01 to the 31st as 31). The date for March 9, 2017 would be recorded as *2017 03 09*. Record the client's date of birth using this same format below the administration date. A client born on November 29, 2012 would be recorded as *2012 11 29*. Now subtract the date of birth from the date of testing. When doing the math, remember that when borrowing from the months column to the days column, you borrow 30 days as that is the typical days in a month; and when borrowing from the years column to the months column, you borrow 12 months as there are 12 months in a year. Start the subtraction with the days column. The following example shows the steps.

1.	State the date of testing	2017 03 09
2.	State the date of birth	−2012 11 29
3.	Subtract starting with the days column	
4.	09 is smaller than 29 so borrow and restate	2017 02 39
		−2012 11 29
		10
5.	Subtract the months column	

6. 02 is smaller than 11 so borrow and restate   2016 14 39
                                                      −2012 11 29
                                                            03 10

7. Subtract the years column
                                                       2016 14 39
                                                      −2012 11 29
                                                         4 03 10

8. The child is 4 years, 3 months, and 10 days old.

9. If the days are 15 or more we round up and add a month, and if the days are under 15 we do not add a month. Thus, we would use the age 4 year 3 months for this client.

In some tests, you begin giving a test at the first test item and administer all the way to the end. There are other tests where the manual instructs you to use the age of the client to determine which item you begin with to administer the testing. Some tests use a basal and/or ceiling item to determine where to begin and end your testing. The basal item is the item where the client has made the specified number of correct responses as stated in the manual (e.g., 3 items correct in a row). You are going to assume all the items before the basal item would have been answered correctly and give him/her credit for those items that occur before the basal. The ceiling item is the test item where the client has made the specified number of errors as stated in the manual, so we stop the testing (e.g., 5 out of 7 items incorrect). The raw score is simply the number of items the client got correct (or in the case of a basal score, the number the client got correct plus the number he was given credit for because they occurred before the basal item). The raw score is a pretty meaningless number until we use it in the comparison tables in the test manual. This process of using the tables in the manual leads us to step four, which is analyzing the results of the testing.

In step four, the clinician compares the client's score to the appropriate norm group tested by the test's author(s) and summarized in table form in the test manual. To determine how the client performed in comparison to his/her peers, the clinician needs the client's age, raw score, and appropriate table(s) in the test manual. By using the tables, the one raw score can be converted into a number of scores that reflect a comparison to the norm group.

A standard score is one commonly reported score. The standard score reflects the client's standing within the bell-shaped curve of a normal distribution; that is, how the score deviates from the mean or average score (add up the set of scores and divide by the number of scores) of the normed comparison group. A normal distribution has half the scores to the left of the mean (average score) of the norm sample (below average) and half the scores to the right of the mean (above average). We use the standard deviation (SD) to describe how our client's score differs from the mean of the norm group. A characteristic of a normal distribution is that 99.7% of the scores are within +/−3 SD of the mean score. A score that is less than 1.5 SD from the mean is considered to be normal or slightly above (to the right) or below (to the left) the normal range. Ninety-two percent of the scores are within this near normal area. The clients that clinicians are concerned about are most often those who are more than 1.5 SD below the mean (–1.5 SD). Only about 4% of the norm group falls in this range. Scores that fall farther below the mean (e.g., –2.5 SD) are considered more severely disordered than those less below the mean (e.g., –1.5 SD). Here is an example to help clarify the use of the standard score. If the test given has a mean of 100 and a standard deviation of 15, then the near normal range (+/–1.5 SD) would be a standard score of 77.5 (100 – 22.5) to a score of 122.5 (100 + 22.5). If a child had a standard score of 70, he/she would be –2 SD from the mean (100 – 30) and typically considered in need of services.

Anyone who has taken a test knows that their score may not reflect their "true" ability. You may have gotten lucky and scored higher than your true ability or may have been influenced by environmental factors, such as a very warm room or lack of sleep, and scored lower than your true ability. Standardized tests authors know this can happen; thus, many tests encourage the clinician to report a confidence interval along with the standard score. This confidence interval is based on the standard error of measurement or the average amount of measurement error across people in the norm group. If the standard error of measurement is both added and subtracted from the score a student receives on a standard test, a range of the student's performance is defined. The clinician can decide to use a relatively smaller range that is more precise, but represents a lower confidence that the student's "true" score was captured (68% confidence interval); or use a broader range that is less precise, but highly likely to include the "true" score (95% or 99% confidence intervals) (Hutchinson, 1996). The 68% confidence interval is typically seen as a meaningful compromise between confidence and precision. The confidence interval information can be found in the test manual and reported on the test record form. This may be reported as the lower limit and upper limits on a test form. The standard score and, less frequently, the confidence interval information are reported in the written report completed by the clinician following an assessment.

While the standard score and confidence interval are commonly used to report the comparison of the client's score to his peers, the percentile rank provides another way to present this information. A percentile rank identifies the percentage of the comparison norm group that scored at or below a given score. In the prior example, the client had a standard score of –2 SD. This would be reflected in a percentile rank of 5% (available in the manual). This client performed better than 5 out of 100 of his peers on this test. The percentile rank can be easily explained to families in a discussion of the test results. Tables may also be provided to convert the raw score into an age-equivalent score. The age-equivalent score represents the average performance of individuals in the test sample of a given chronological age. Thus, a child who has a tabled age equivalent score of 3 years 2 months obtained a raw score that was the average raw score from the sample of children at that age. Age-equivalent scores do not account for differences in developmental rate across ages, and compared to the other derived measures, are less likely to be stable estimates of the child's skill. While on the face, age-equivalent measures appear easy to understand; however, they are in fact problematic and are not recommended for making placement decisions (Silverlake, 1999).

The last step in this process is reporting the results both verbally to the client and family and in writing in the diagnostic report. In general, when reporting results, the clinician identifies the area(s) assessed, the name and a brief description of the test used, the results of the testing, what the results mean in terms of a disorder being present or absent, and, if present, the severity of the disorder. Areas of relative strength and weakness should also be stated.

Why

The standardized test is an objective measure that provides a comparison of the client's results to that of his/her peers. They are widely used for enrollment purposes. Standardized tests should always be accompanied by of information obtained by interviews, samples, dynamic assessment, and structured interactions to provide a more holistic view of the client's skills and limitations.

When

Most standardized testing is done prior to enrollment in treatment. Additional standardized testing may be done for yearly reevaluation or dismissal.

Where

Standardized testing is most typically done in a quiet environment with only the clinician and client present. When parents or caregivers are present, the clinician will set the stage to decrease the distraction or likelihood of others influencing the client's responses.

How

It is important for the clinician to be prepared before testing, accurate and observant during testing, and truthful, timely, and clear in reporting results following testing.

Top 10 Terms

Basal
Ceiling
Confidence interval
Normal bell-shaped curve
Percentile rank
Practice items
Raw score
Standard deviation
Standard score
Test items

Chapter Tips

1. Always fill out the test record form completely and accurately. A partially completed form is of limited value. Good record keeping is vital and will be essential if legal or ethical questions are raised in the future.

2. Make note of other observations you have during the standardized testing. A child who repeats back the instructions you provide during testing or asks for feedback after testing has provided the observant clinician with important prognostic information.

3. Commercially available tests set up their comparison tables differently. The manual will often have an example of how the test form is to be completed. If you are unable to understand how to use the comparison table(s), go to the example and use the example client's age and raw score to see where comparison scores are in the table(s). In other words, take the example and work backward until you understand how the information was determined.

Activities

5–1. Given the following dates, determine the client's, Ann, age used in administering and scoring a test.

Date clinician is writing report = April 1, 2017

Date clinician gave test = March 26, 2017

Client's date of birth = May 2, 2011

Clinician's date of birth = June 8, 1994

5–2. Given the following dates, determine the client's, Bill, age used in administering and scoring a test.

Date clinician is writing report = February 1, 2018

Date clinician gave test = January 28, 2018

Client's date of birth = November 10, 1998

5–3. Child A is 4 years old, Child B is 6 years old, and Child C is 8 years old. They all score a raw score of 45 on a standardized test. Can you make any definitive statement about each of their abilities? What else do you need to analyze their results?

_____

_____

_____

_____

5–4. Explain to a parent what a score in the 15th percentile means.

Answers to Activities

5–1.

	2017	3	26	= 2016	15	26
−	2011	5	2	− 2011	5	2
				5	10	24 = 5 years 1 months

5–2.

	2017	1	28	= 2017	13	28
−	1998	11	10	− 1998	11	10
				19	2	18 = 19 years 3 months

5–3. A raw score alone does not provide useful information. You need to have the tables in the manual to determine their standard scores and confidence interval or their percentile ranks. It is possible a raw score of 45 puts all the children above the mean. It is just as likely that it would place all the children below the mean. A raw score alone is just not enough information.

5–4. Your child scored in the 15th percentile on this standardized test. This means that your child performed better than 15 of 100 same-aged peers who took this exam.

Wrap-Up

1. Complete Table 5–1. In column 1, list five specific pieces of information you expect to find in a test manual. In column 2, locate and state those pieces of information from an available test manual including page numbers from the manual. In the starred (*) rows of the table, identify two additional pieces of information you did not have in your list that were in the manual.

2. Describe a scenario where a clinician might choose to select a language test with a broad focus and a second scenario where a language test with a narrow focus would be appropriate.

Table 5–1. Five Specific Pieces of Information Expected to Be Found in a Test Manual

Test Name:_____

Information You Expect to Find	Specific Information Found Including Page Number from the Manual
1.	
2.	
3.	
4.	
5.	
*	
*	

Scenario #1—broad focus

_____
_____
_____
_____

Scenario #2—narrow focus

_____
_____
_____
_____

3. Why do you think a test—such as an articulation test—does not use a basal or ceiling, but requires the entire test be administered to each client?

_____
_____
_____
_____

4. You have a budget of $500 to purchase one or more tests for your practice. List five factors you would consider in making your selections.

Factor 1 = _____

Factor 2 = _____

Factor 3 = _____

Factor 4 = _____

Factor 5 = _____

References

Fulcher-Rood, K., Castilla-Earls, A. P., & Higginbotham, J. (2018). School-based speech-language pathologists' perspectives on diagnostic decision making. *American Journal of Speech-Language Pathology, 27,* 796–814. doi:10-1044/2018-AJSLP-16-0121

Hegde, M. N., & Pomaville, F. (2013). *Assessment of communication disorders in children resources and protocols* (2nd ed.). San Diego, CA: Plural Publishing Inc.

Hutchinson, T. A. (1996). What to look for in the technical manual: Twenty questions for users. *Language, Speech and Hearing Services in Schools, 27,* 109–121.

McCauley, R. J., & Swisher, L. (1984). Psychometric review of language and articulation tests for preschool children. *Journal of Speech and Hearing Disorders, 49,* 34–42.

Plante, E. (1996). Observing and interpreting behavior: An introduction to the clinical forum. *Language, Speech, and Hearing Services in Schools, 27,* 99–101.

Silverlake, A. C. (1999). *Comprehending test manuals.* Los Angeles, CA: Pyrczak.

CHAPTER 6

Statistical Basis

Who

Clinicians need some understanding of mathematical processes and statistics in order to be good evaluators. This chapter will look at the basic math concepts and skills a clinician should understand to make it easier to read test manuals and provide accurate testing and scoring methods. For a more thorough explanation of how to comprehend test manuals, the authors refer you to *Comprehending Test Manuals* (Silverlake, 1999). It is also important to understand the terms and information you will be reporting so that clinicians can explain the results of testing to parents or others who may not be familiar with the testing process and results. As Lewis (2015) states, "We forget that many of the statistical terms speech-language pathologists and educators use regularly remain a mystery to most." The more comfortable a clinician is with the terms used in testing, the easier it is to explain the test and results.

What

Certain terms should be very familiar to a clinician in order to make sure the clinician is able to accurately read a test manual, perform the assessment, score the assessment, and report the information. The ability to read charts is also necessary for clinicians. Before clinicians even get to the point of giving an assessment, they should be well aware of the sensitivity and specificity of the test they are interested in giving. The validity of a test (or how well the test accurately measures what it is supposed to) should be reviewed to make sure the clinician is using a good tool to identify a problem area (Parikh, Mathai, Parikh, Chandra Sekhar, & Thomas, 2008). Hutchinson (1996) suggests a simple and important question regarding validity, "Is the purpose of this test explicitly stated?" (p. 112). Validity is measured by sensitivity and specificity. Sensitivity is the ability of the test to correctly classify an individual as "disordered" (Parikh et al., 2008). Specificity is the ability of a test to correctly identify an individual to be within normal limits. This chapter will focus on terms and charts to ensure a clinician is prepared for the assessment process.

The following terms should be very familiar to a clinician:

- Mean: The average. Mean is determined by adding a set of scores together and dividing the total by the number of scores. For example, if five students had the following scores: 72, 84, 85, 88, 90, the mean would be 83.8.

- Median: The middle score. This is determined by putting the scores in numerical order from least to greatest. The middle score would be the score where half of the testers scored lower and half the testers scored higher. For example, if seven students had the following scores: 58, 64, 70, 75, 80, 86, 100, the median would be 75.
- N: This is typically the number of tests given. N is needed to determine mean and median.
- Standard Deviation: A measure of variability or spread. This is used to determine how much an individual's score differs from the mean of the comparison, or norm, group.
- Correlation: How two variables move in sync with one another. For correlation, a + 1 indicates they move in sync perfectly, a – 1 means they move opposite one another perfectly, and 0 means that changing one does not change the other. For example, if you take this made up scenario—running more and eating more carbohydrates—a + 1 correlation would mean the more you run, the more carbohydrates you eat. A – 1 correlation would mean the more you run, the fewer carbs you eat. And a 0 correlation would mean the two have no effect on one another.
- Raw Score: The number of questions answered correctly.
- Reliability: The ability to reproduce the results repeatedly.
- Validity: How much meaning can be placed on a set of test results.
- Percentile rank: The percentage of people scoring at or below a particular score.

When looking at charts it is most important for the clinician to know what data they are interpreting. A chart will have a description to help the clinician know what information the chart contains. A clinician should make themselves familiar with many different types of charts. Some charts will have numerical values, while others may use bar graphs or bell curves. In a test manual, a clinician should be able to locate charts to help determine the reliability and validity of that particular test as well as charts that will help the clinician score the test results. Table 6–1 is a chart that shows normative data of a test. Table 6–2 is a chart that would help the clinician transfer a raw score to a standard score.

Table 6–1. Standardization Sample by Age

Age Group	Total
2.0 – 2.6	103
2.7 – 2.11	99
3.0 – 3.6	107
3.7 – 3.11	104
4.0 – 4.6	97
4.7 – 5.0	105

Table 6–2. Raw Score to Standard Score Conversion Chart

Raw Score	Standard Score
25	80
26	81
27	82
28	83
29	84
30	85

Why

Clinicians will need to be able to complete certain mathematical concepts/equations and/or read charts to determine information such as chronological age, standard scores, standard deviations, reliability, validity, percentile rank, and occurrence of phonological processes.

When

Clinicians will need to review test manuals prior to completing the evaluation. A clinician should become familiar with test instructions, what the test is capable of determining, what scores will be given, how to score the results, and how to interpret the results.

Scoring will not be completed until the evaluation is finished; however, a clinician will need to know information such as chronological age prior to determining appropriate assessment tools. Once the evaluation is complete, a clinician will score the tests and interpret those results. If a standardized assessment tool is not given as specified in the manual, the clinician will not be able to use the test scores and will instead have to use the results as more narrative information.

Where

Most often, the statistical information will be done by the clinician without the client present. This could be in an office or clinical setting. There will be times when a clinician may need to complete some preliminary calculations during a test to determine if a test should be continued. Often, the clinician will want to provide the client and/or caretakers with basic information prior to them leaving the assessment session. While clinicians are not often expected to complete the entire scoring process during the evaluation session, it is often helpful to be able to give some information on next steps at the end of an evaluation.

How

Determining chronological age has been covered in previous chapters, but a quick review is also provided here. To determine chronological age, the clinician will need the patient's date of birth and the date of testing. The clinician will subtract the date of testing from the date of birth (organized as year, month, and day). Remember, if the date of birth is not easily subtracted from the date of testing, subtraction with borrowing must occur. For months, use 12; for days, use 30. Because many score charts are used with year/month only (e.g., 2.9 is 2 years, 9 months), when the days are determined, you may need to adjust the months. If the days are between 0 and 15, we use the month number we calculated; whereas, if the days are more than 15, we add one month to the number that was calculated (2 years, 8 months, and 17 days would calculate to 2.9). An example of calculating chronological age follows:

Date of birth: 11/24/1980
Date of evaluation: 09/26/2017
Equation:
    2016/21
    ~~2017~~/09/26
    −1980/11/24
= 26 years, 10 months, 2 days—for most charts you would use 26.10 (26 years, 10 months)

When reading tables or charts, a clinician must know what data is being determined. Most often, tables will have keys or legends that will let you know what data is included in the table or chart. Heading information can also help the clinician know how the table helps with scoring data or determining how the test was normed. Clinicians will often see the < or > signs when reading tables. Clinicians are reminded that when the value on the left is less than the value on the right, the < (less than) sign is used. When the value on the left is greater than the value on the right, the > (greater than) sign is used. Using Table 6–3, you will see that a raw score of 50 gives a standard score of less than 45 and a percentile rank of less than 1.

When determining the existence of phonological processes, a clinician will typically determine how often in speech the process is being used. This is often confusing to

Table 6–3. Raw Score Conversion Chart for Standard Score and Percentile Rank

Raw Score	Standard Score	Percentile Rank
55	49	3
54	48	2
53	47	2
52	46	1
51	<45	1
50	<45	<1

clinicians as it could be written in terms of how often it occurs (90% of the time: so 90% of the time the child is using this particular process). When clinicians write goals for phonological processes, they can be written as reducing the occurrence (typically we use 40% as the goal: so we want the child to get below 40% use) or increasing the correct production. When assessing a phonological process, the higher the percentage of use, the more difficult it will likely be to understand the connected speech (or sometimes even individual words) of the child.

Top 10 Terms

Mean

Median

Standard deviation

Reliability

Validity

Correlation

Percentile rank

Raw scores

Chronological age

Sensitivity

Chapter Tips

1. Making sure a test is valid is the first step in determining what evaluation tool will be used to assess a patient. Clinicians should be familiar with basic terms and charts in order to accurately read test manuals as well as score tests.
2. Prior to determining what test is appropriate for the patient, the clinician should calculate chronological age and areas needed for assessment.
3. A clinician should be prepared to complete some preliminary calculations or determinations at the end of an assessment session in order to discuss the overall results with the patient and/or caregivers.

Activities

6–1. Using he chart in Table 6–3, determine the percentile rank and standard score for a patient who had a raw score of 53.

6–2. Using the chart in Table 6–1, determine the number of children aged 3.3 who were given the test as part of the normative process.

6-3. Using the chart in Table 6-2, determine the standard score if the raw score is 28.

6-4. Determine the median and mode of the following sets of information:

a. Scores = 24, 56, 42, 38, 27
Mean: _____
Median: _____

b. Scores = 76, 77, 78, 82, 79, 85, 83, 88, 90
Mean: _____
Median: _____

c. Scores = 10, 14, 17, 22, 25, 32, 37
Mean: _____
Median: _____

6-5. Determine the correct symbol use for the information given.

a. H is less than five: H ____ 5

b. Three is less than H: H ____ 3

Answers to Activities

6-1. Standard score = 47; percentile rank = 2
6-2. $N = 107$
6-3. Standard score = 83
6-4. a. Mean = 37.4; Median = 38
b. Mean = 82; Median = 82
c. Mean = 22.43; Median = 22
6-5. a. <
b. >

Wrap-Up

1. In the space provided, make your own chart to depict raw score, standard score, and percentile rank for a given set of data. Draw a normal curve and identify the relationship of mean and median in a normal curve using the data from your chart.

Chapter 6 • Statistical Basis 59

2. Find and compare two test manuals for tests that are typically given in your clinic setting. Answer the following questions:

   1. What are the tests? What areas do they test?

   _____
   _____
   _____
   _____
   _____

   2. What are the age ranges for the tests?

   _____
   _____

   3. How were the tests normed? Are there charts showing normative data? What normative data is given?

   _____
   _____

4. Do the tests use percentile rank, age equivalents, and/or other information?

5. What charts or information are helpful when scoring these tests? Give a description of the information obtained by comparing a patient's responses to these charts.

References

Hutchinson, T. A. (1996). What to look for in the technical manual. *Language, Speech, and Hearing Services in the Schools, 27*(2), 109–121.

Lewis, K. S. (2015, September 29). *How to share stats with parents*. Retrieved from https://blog.asha.org/2015/09/29/sharing-stats-with-parents/

Parikh, R., Mathai, A., Parikh, S., Chandra Sekhar, G., & Thomas, R. (2008). Understanding and using sensitivity, specificity and predictive values. *Indian Journal of Ophthalmology, 56*(1), 45–50.

Silverlake, A. C. (1999). *Comprehending test manuals: A guide and workbook*. Los Angeles, CA: Pyrczak Pub.

CHAPTER 7

Dynamic Assessment

Who

Dynamic assessment is appropriate for most evaluations because it provides information to augment other testing and is useful in planning remediation techniques that are effective for a specific client. A standardized test can tell you how the client performs compared to his/her peers or the severity level of the disorder, but additional information is needed before a clinician will know how to commence treatment. Dynamic assessment is especially useful with children with significant disorders as the best therapeutic approach to use will vary greatly depending on the individual and their ideal learning needs (Binger, Kent-Walsh, & King, 2017). Assessment that goes beyond standardized tests is also used for culturally diverse clients who may have different prior environmental or language experiences (Ebert & Pham, 2017; Engel de Abreu, Baldassi, Puglisi, & Befi-Lopes, 2013). Language sample analysis and dynamic assessment have been found to be effective in the identification of language impairment in bilingual children (De Lamo White & Jin, 2011). There is an art to being good at dynamic assessment that develops with practice.

What

Dynamic assessment is a unique nonstatic examination of a client's potential for learning via a quick minitrial therapy technique. It varies client to client, situation to situation, and clinician to clinician. It requires flexibility and thoughtful consideration on the part of the clinician. No one procedure fits every situation. "Test-teach-test," degree of examiner effort, and client explanation are among the ways used to perform dynamic assessment.

Sometimes a structured interaction is set up by the clinician to gauge what works for this client. A test-teach-test format is a common form of dynamic assessment. Stimulability testing in articulation assessment is a classic example of the test-teach-test format that is widely used. When an error has been made in a sound in the target word on the standardized articulation test, the clinician follows up with a dynamic assessment termed stimulability testing. The clinician will elicit the sound in isolation following a model, modification of another sound, placement cues, and/or look at the clinician or look in the mirror reminder. If the child is successful with cues at the isolation level, the linguistic complexity is increased to syllable, then words, then phrases, and then sentences. If one cue is not helpful, then other cues or a combination of cues may be attempted. Thus, the dynamic assessment adds information on degree and type of cueing that is most supportive for a particular client and also linguistic level where treatment should initially focus.

Sometimes the clinician uses dynamic assessment as a gauge if they are planning to remediate at an appropriate difficulty level or use a particular strategy. Here, they would provide a task, demonstrate a strategy for approaching the task, and discuss the problem, strategy, and solution. Then, a second, similar task would be given and the client's ability to transfer the previous strategy to a new but similar task would be evaluated. Ultimately, the clinician could gauge the amount of examiner effort needed for the client to be successful at the task on a 3- or 5-point scale. A clinician rating of effort that was required to stimulate or cue the client to make a correct response provides insight into the client's readiness for a specific treatment technique or level. Peña (2000) used a Modifiability Scale that included a rating of perceived examiner effort, child responsivity (attention, planning, self-regulation, motivation), and transfer. For examiner effort, a score of 0 indicated extreme examiner effort, 1 indicated high–moderate effort, 2 indicated moderate effort, and 3 indicated slight effort. For child responsivity, a score of 0 indicated no responsivity at all, 1 indicated slight responsivity, 2 indicated moderate responsivity, and 3 indicated high responsivity. For the transfer scale, 0 was low, 1 was moderate, and 2 was high. In general, the more precisely the scale scores are defined and described, the more reliable the score will be across evaluators. If you use or develop a rating scale in your dynamic assessment, make sure you identify how each score is distinct.

Asking a client to explain their answers can serve a useful part of the dynamic process. For example, the clinician gave the client a dynamic receptive task (child manipulated items as directed instead of providing verbalized or written answers) of separating picture cards of toys, food, and clothing into piles or categories after he scored low on categorization on a standardized test. In this case, the 4-year-old child separated them into three piles but no clear semantic categories seemed to be identified. Rather than just noting the client was unsuccessful with the task, the clinician questioned the child as to why he separated them in this particular way. The child revealed his separation was based on whether the circle vowel "o" or dot above an "i" was present in the small printed word on the bottom of the card. Further examination revealed that the child was hyperlexic or had an excessive focus on print. This information lead to a referral to a psychologist for additional testing and identification of the need for careful consideration in material selection for the remediation process.

Why

While standardized tests compare the client to his/her same aged peers, dynamic assessments focus on the unique characteristics of the individual as they relate to possible remediation efforts. For populations where standardized tests are not reliable and or valid, such as clients who are culturally or linguistically diverse, dynamic assessment measures can provide helpful information for distinguishing between a language difference and a language disorder. Dynamic assessment allows the clinician to consider how a child approaches learning language and not merely what language knowledge a child already possesses. Dynamic assessment along with multiple observations, language samples, interviews, and questionnaires are components of the assessment of children learning English as a second language (Harten, 2011).

When

Dynamic assessment can be used at any time, but is most common immediately following a standard assessment and prior to remediation being implemented; or in the case of culturally and linguistically diverse individuals, as an alternative or supplement to a standardized assessment.

Where

Dynamic assessment is usually done in a one-on-one session with client and clinician. Remember, in dynamic assessment we are interested in this individual's learning level and selection of appropriate learning strategies.

How

While dynamic assessment requires flexibility, it should begin with an *organized plan* of (a) concept to be assessed (what question[s] are you trying to answer or what content area you are exploring); (b) steps you will use to assess including a discussion with the client as to the reasons for his/her response (perhaps a technique you wish to try or a script you plan to follow); (c) how you will analyze the results (change in test-teach-test format or perhaps a cueing hierarchy rating or a measure of examiner effort); and (d) recommendations for interpreting the results perhaps in a decision tree format (if this happens, then this is the recommendation). Larson and McKinley (2007) propose this type of organized plan as Specific Intervention Methods and include the components of mediation and bridging questions within the plan. Mediation questions focus the learner on the task or strategy to use, while bridging questions focus the learner on where and when the strategy might be used in their daily life. An example of a mediating question would be, "What do we focus on when separating items into categories—the spelling of the word or the function of the item?" A bridging question would be, "How would finding an apple in a grocery store be easier if we knew it belonged to the category of fruit and not the category of dairy?"

There is no one right way to plan a dynamic assessment. The example provided in Figure 7–1 is an organized plan that *could* be developed before seeing a kindergarten-aged child whose teacher reports that he calls items by names that reflect the item's function (e.g., "beater" for "heart"). This has resulted in academic errors when a picture of a "heart" is circled as a "B" word and a picture of a "finger" is circled as a "P" word. A specialty standardized test for word finding difficulties identified this child as a "fast and inaccurate namer." Figure 7–1 presents a dynamic assessment plan for this child.

Dynamic Assessment Plan

Client Name: <u>Carrie Kinder</u>　　　　　Age: <u>5 years 2 months</u>　　　　　Date: <u>4/25/2018</u>

History/file: No family history of word finding difficulties were noted.

Interview: Teacher reported that she called items by names that reflect the items function (e.g. "beater" for "heart") which leads to academic errors. Mrs. Kinder reported that Carrie frequently makes up her own words but understands what is said to her.

Test results: Carrie scored a Word Finding Index of 70 on <u>Test of Word Finding–third edition</u> (TWF-3) which indicated a likely word finding problem that requires remediation. She was further identified as a "fast and inaccurate namer" meaning she had a quick response time and many errors in naming nouns whose names she recognized receptively.

Observation: A 20-minute classroom observation during self-selected center time revealed Carrie participated in all tasks at an appropriate level. She demonstrated minimal frustration when asked to repeat or expand her answers. Her peers appeared to seek interactions with Carrie.

Steps to follow	Plan for client	Results
a) concept to be assessed (what question(s) are you trying to answer or what content area are you exploring)	Area = word finding; Would slowing her response time result in higher accuracy? Does child recognize strategies that improve her naming accuracy?	
b) steps you will use to assess including a discussion with the client as to the reasons for his response (perhaps a technique you wish to try or a script you plan to follow)	*Test-teach-test format*: Present 10 pictures of common items and ask her to name (test); teach her to look at/think about the picture but not give the name until the clinician points at her (5 second delay). About a 5-minute mini-teaching lesson using a second set of pictures to practice waiting before naming (teach). Represent the 10 original pictures (test). *Client explanation*: Ask her about her experience in naming object, what works for her, how it felt to wait before responding, what happens when we call something by the wrong name etc.	
c) how you will analyze the results (change in test-teach-test format or perhaps a cueing hierarchy rating or a measure of examiner effort)	Comparison of accuracy (test vs. re-test) in naming based on increased wait time. Client awareness of naming difficulty and thought about strategies could be rated from 1–3 (1 = no awareness; 2 = awareness but no idea what works to help; 3 = very aware and has suggestions of what helps or hurts recall).	
d) recommendations for interpreting the results (if this happens then this is the recommendation)	If change occurs due to longer wait time recommend this as a strategy for remediation. If no change made due to wait time, consider a 2nd strategy (e.g. making 2 meaningful sentences about each item prior to naming) for test-teach-test format. Perhaps set up a trial using a technique the client identified as useful.	

Summary of results/recommendations from dynamic assessment:

Figure 7–1. Dynamic assessment plan for a child.

Top 10 Terms

Bridging question
Client explanation
Dynamic assessment
Receptive task
Examiner effort
Mediating question
Semantic category
Static assessment
Stimulability testing
Test-teach-test

Chapter Tips

1. Do not use the items from the standardized test as your material or targets for a dynamic assessment. Using the standardized test material to teach results in bias, if the test were ever used again with this client. Instead of using the materials or test items from the standardized test, gather items based on the **concept** to be addressed.

2. Mediating and bridging questions are not limited to use in dynamic assessment. They should be used throughout the remediation process to encourage strategy learning and generalization.

3. Just a reminder that when assessing a child who is an English Language Learner, the assessment must include both languages.

Activities

7–1. Identify whether the following questions are seeking to mediate (focus on the task) or bridge (focus on life applications) by putting the correct term before each item.

1. _____ We have practiced taking smaller bites and sitting up straight when eating to help prevent choking during meals. Where do you think is the best place for you to eat lunch when you go home next week?

2. _____ This sentence has three /m/ sounds in it. Put your finger on each /m/ word. Now, let's read the sentences using good sounds.

3. _____ We have practiced two fluency enhancing strategies. Can you demonstrate them both before we end our session today?

4. _____ When you answer the phone this evening, which of the fluency enhancing strategies will you use?

5. _____ You read that passage using all correct /r/ sounds. When during your day do you think it would be important to read out loud using correct /r/ sounds?

7–2. In stimulability testing in articulation assessment, the clinician will elicit the sound using one or more of the following cues: (a) following a model, (b) after providing a placement cue, (c) as a modification of another sound, and/or (d) reminder to look at the clinician or in the mirror. Identify which of the four cues each of the following statements describes. More than one cue might be present in the description. List all that are present.

1. _____ Look and listen to me. Say /ki/.

2. _____ Close your teeth and do not let you tongue between your teeth.

3. _____ Start by making an /l/ sound and keep moving your tongue along the top of your mouth until it sounds like this, /r/.

4. _____ Look in the mirror and say the word three times.

5. _____ Put your tongue on the bump behind your teeth.

Answers to Activities

7–1

1. Bridging
2. Mediating
3. Mediating
4. Bridging
5. Bridging

7–2

1. (a) model and d) look
2. (b) placement
3. (c) modification of another sound, b) placement, and a) model
4. (d) mirror
5. (b) placement

Wrap-Up

1. Describe what practices you see as the "art" of assessment and what practices you see as the "science" of assessment.

Art =

_____
_____

Science =

_____
_____

2. Think of an experience you have had teaching someone a skill. Perhaps you have taught a family member how to use something on their phone or computer. Write a short paragraph describing what you taught and how it went.

_____
_____
_____
_____

3. Regarding the experience in #2, think about the effort you put into having that person learn that skill. Devise descriptors to define the effort to another person and explain how to use your scale. Provide a description for a score of 1, 2, 3, 4, and 5.

Score of 1 =

_____
_____

Score of 2 =

_____
_____

Score of 3 =

_____
_____

Score of 4 =

_____
_____

Score of 5 =

4. If I were testing a child whose culture had a greater comfort level in a long silence after a question than is typical in the United States, what might I erroneously conclude?

5. Research and state a specific cultural difference that could impact your assessment process.

References

Binger, C., Kent-Walsh, J., & King, M. (2017). Dynamic assessment for 3- and 4-year-old children who use augmentative and alternative communication: Evaluating expressive syntax. *Journal of Speech, Language, and Hearing Research, 60,* 1946–1958.

DeLamo White, C., & Jin, L. (2011). Evaluation of speech language assessment approaches with bilingual children. *International Journal of Language and Communication Disorders, 46*(6), 613–627. doi: 10.111/j.1460-6984.2011.00049x

Ebert, K. D., & Pham, G. (2017). Synthesizing information from language samples and standardized tests in school-age bilingual assessment. *Language Speech, and Hearing Services in School, 48,* 42–55.

German, D. J. (2014). Test of word finding (3rd ed.; TWF-3) [Assessment instrument]. Austin, TX: Pro-Ed.

Harten, A. C. (2011). Multicultural issues in assessment and intervention. In R. B. Hoodin (Ed.), *Intervention in child language disorders* (pp. 125–150). Sudbury, MA: Jones & Bartlett.

Larson, V.L. (2007). Communication solutions for older students assessment and intervention strategies. Greenville, SC: Thinking Publications.

Peña, E. (2000). Measurement of modifiability in children from culturally and linguistically diverse backgrounds. *Communication Disorders Quarterly, 21*(2), 87–97.

CHAPTER 8

Observation

Who

Every diagnostician must be a competent observer. Observation is important in the initial assessment and remains important through ongoing diagnostic treatment and into the dismissal process. Clinicians always have their "eyes and ears open." They are watching for things such as the impact of situational factors, partner influences, complexity of language interactions, changes in skill levels, generalization within and beyond the therapy session, and additional areas for referral. While observation is always important, it is relied on to an even higher degree when assessing individuals who are culturally diverse or demonstrate a severe disability. Cultural bias of tests and unfamiliar procedures make observations of a variety of situations, partners, and languages essential.

What

Observation is the act of paying attention to the factor or factors about which you are gathering information. Observations in behavioral terms should include three components: the antecedent events (things that happened before the behavior), the behavior itself, and the consequences (things that occurred after the behavior) (Richards, Taylor, Ramasamy, & Richards, 1999). By having information on all three components, the clinician can better plan treatment to increase or decrease the behavior. If we were observing swallowing behavior, we would want information on the consistency and amount of the food or liquid as well as the posture of the patient as antecedent events. The swallow itself would be described as the behavior of interest. Finally, consequences such as cough, wet voice, or regurgitations following the swallow would also be important to report.

Information on behaviors can be generally reported as "appearances" or specifically reported by a "count" of the occurrence of a behavior in a given period. Based on observation, a report may state in a general fashion, "voice and fluency appeared within the normal range" or "articulation errors appeared consistent with those noted in the formal test of articulation production." A specific count of a behavior may be reported as, "five occurrences of whole-word repetition occurred in a 10-min play observation" or "no occurrences of interactive play were observed during the 20-min recess." While observing sounds easy, in reality, it is a hard thing to do well.

The work by Simons and Chabris (1999) titled *Gorillas in Our Midst: Sustained Inattentional Blindness for Dynamic Events* demonstrated how people viewing a video of players passing a ball around may fail to see the unusual appearance of a gorilla entering the scene because unexpected events may be overlooked. There are a number of similar examples available on YouTube that you might wish to view with friends and then gather data on which of your friends "sees the gorilla." It seems evident that focus on one behavior may affect the observation of other unexpected elements. While there is no one way to ensure that you will view all the relevant facts, multiple observations across several situations is suggested. Also, checking in with other sources (parents, other team members, and the clients themselves) as to the accuracy of your observations will add credibility to your observations. Including examples of behaviors observed as part of the report also aids the reader of the report in understanding and valuing your conclusions.

Why

Two common functions of observations in evaluation are a *confirmation-refining function* and a *screening function*. In any diagnostic evaluation, there will be components of the communication process that will be observed and reported in conjunction with reporting more formal measures. In such cases, observations may confirm or lead to refining the outcomes of the test findings in more authentic communication interactions. The question of how the identified deficits play out in real speaking, reading, writing, and/or listening events is critical. Thus, most initial evaluations will have an interaction/observation component included before a diagnosis is rendered. Once a client is in therapy, observations are commonly reported as subjective information within each session note. Before a dismissal is recommended, the clinician again considers what they have observed of actual communication skills. Damico (1988) presented a compelling argument for not only relying on test results that fragment language skills into components parts, but rather viewing them within a context of social and environmental factors. The case he presented of a child dismissed from therapy then several years later reevaluated by the same clinician and identified with a significant language impairment highlights several factors that can lead to misdiagnosis, including the failure to put language into a broader context.

The screening function of observations typically occur in those speech, language, and swallowing areas that are not of primary focus in the evaluation. If the primary diagnostic questions to be addressed concern the client's language abilities, then the secondary areas such as voice and fluency may be assessed exclusively through observation. If the primary questions concern the client's fluency, then secondary areas such as voice, articulation, and language may be examined through observation. If this observation leads to concerns in any of these areas, then additional formal measures of the selected area will be added or recommended for future testing. Thus, in these instances, observation served as a screening function.

When

There is no right or wrong time for observation of communication skills. A clinician should always be a vigilant observer.

Where

Several shorter observations, especially in a variety of places and situations and with a variety of partners, is more advantageous than one longer observation. The ease of videotaping via smart phones can facilitate families in providing taped samples for clinicians to use to gain observation information in places they might not typically have access. There is no part of the diagnostic process where being observant is not important. In general, the more natural, real-life place(s) and situation(s) in which the observation(s) occurs, the better.

How

There is no one right way to do or organize information from an observation. Videotaping or audiotaping allows for multiple viewings of the sample, which can be useful. When observations are not taped, the clinician may take field notes on what they are observing by

---

Specified Focus Observation Form

Name of client: _____ Date: _____
Purpose of observation/Questions to be answered by the observation: _____

Place: _____ Individuals present: _____
Length of observation: _____
General description of procedure(s) used: _____

Observer: _____

Before you begin, list characteristics you want to gather information about in the first column.

After the observation, describe examples of the behavior in columns 2 and 3. Next in column 3, form conclusions about your characteristic–would you rate it as too much, normal, or too little?

Finally summarize your observation at the bottom of the form.

Characteristic	Example	Example	Too much Normal Too Little

Summary of observation(s):

Figure 8–1. Example of a Specified Focus Observation Form.

```
Open Focus Observation Form

Name of client: _____ Date:_____
Purpose of observation/Questions to be answered by the observation: _____
_____
Place: _____ Individuals present: _____
Length of observation: _____
General description of procedure(s) used: _____
_____
Observer: _____

Record your observations in the space below.  Summarize your findings at the bottom of the form.




Summary of observation:

```

Figure 8–2. Example of an Open Focus Observation Form.

noting things such as what was said or done, the participants, and the activity, or the clinician may note examples of focus behaviors. Developing a form to help you organize your observational information can be helpful. Two such forms are provided in Figure 8–1 and 8–2. The Specified Focus Observation Form is organized around predetermined characteristics of importance, while the Open Focus Observation Form is more a blank page approach. If the clinician chooses to use the Specified Focus Form, he/she should list characteristics typically of interest prior to the observation. Both approaches to observation have advantages and disadvantages.

Top 10 Terms

Antecedent events

Confirmation-refining function

Conclusions

Consequences

Observation

Observations as "appearances"

Observations as "count"

Open focus observation

Screening function
Specific focus observation

Chapter Tips

1. Examples of specific behaviors observed are often interwoven with conclusions the observer has made. These are different things. Behaviors are evident to all seeing them, while conclusions are the interpretation of the behavior observed. Someone may be observed crying, while observers may have differing opinions as to whether the crying is expressing relief, frustration, or sadness. Examples of specific behaviors observed are descriptions of instances that are used to illustrate the conclusions the clinician has reached. Terms such as reached, said, read, pointed, identified, and smiled are terms used to specify a behavior, while enthusiastic, understood, comprehended, and expected are conclusions reached by the clinician based on the observation.
2. Remember to confirm your observation with others; observe across settings, situations, and partners; and provide clear examples of your observations.
3. The American Speech-Language-Hearing Association (ASHA) requires that 25 hr of clinical observation be completed as part of the required 400 hr clinical experience (American Speech-Language-Hearing Association, n.d.). These hours are an excellent time for preprofessionals to develop their observational skills not only about characteristics of a disorder, but also about many important features of the clinical situation (Hall, 2016). Take full advantage of your clinical observations to begin to develop these crucial skills.

Activities

8–1. The following is an excerpt from a diagnostic report summarizing the observations of a 4-year-old child's language skills. Identify whether each listed item is a specific behavior observed or a conclusion drawn by putting an O for observed behavior, a C for conclusion, or O & C for both an observable behavior and conclusion given before each item.

Symbolic Use: Johnny was able to communicate using actions, gestures, and some vocalizations that pertained to immediate needs or interests in the environment. During his interaction with the graduate clinician, he was observed pushing away books when bored and using symbol play by pretending to drink from a cup. In addition, when he was ready to leave, he pointed toward the door and waved good-bye. This data reflects that he is at the nonsymbolic level.

1. ____ Johnny was able to communicate using actions, gestures, and some vocalizations that pertained to immediate needs or interests in the environment.
2. ____ He was observed pushing away books when bored.

3. ____ He was observed using symbol play by pretending to drink from a cup.
4. ____ In addition, when he was ready to leave he pointed toward the door.
5. ____ Johnny waved good-bye.
6. ____ This data reflects that he is at the nonsymbolic level.

8–2. Match the list of characteristics a clinician might put in the characteristic column on the Specific Observation Form with the disorder the list best represents. A list of disorders to choose from is provided in the following Disorders Word Bank.

1. _____ syntax, morphology, semantics, phonology, pragmatics
2. _____ partner influence, gestures, eye contact, turn taking
3. _____ pitch, nasal resonance, loudness, quality, and breathing
4. _____ addition, substitutions, omissions, distortions, process errors, syllable structure, reaction when asked to correct, occurrence of self-correction
5. _____ attention, memory, sequencing, problem solving
6. _____ repetitions, prolongations, silent pauses, circumlocutions, secondary symptoms, rate
7. _____ leans in, watches lips, high frequency sound errors, asks for repetitions
8. _____ cough, drooling, wet voice, inability to maintain lip closure, food/liquid remaining in oral cavity after swallow, food/liquid leaking from nasal cavity when eating/drinking
9. _____ symbol use, communication aids, modalities, fine motor, matching skill

Disorders Word Bank—select from the following disorders to fill in the blanks

Cognitive aspects of communication

Communication modalities

Fluency

Hearing

Receptive/expressive language

Speech sound/articulation

Social aspects of communication

Swallowing

Voice and resonance

Answers to Activities

8–1

1. O & C
2. O & C
3. O & C
4. O & C
5. O
6. C

8–2

1. Receptive/expressive language
2. Social aspects
3. Voice and resonance
4. Speech sound/articulation
5. Cognitive aspects of communication
6. Fluency
7. Hearing
8. Swallowing
9. Communication modalities

Wrap-Up

1. Two observation forms are provided for your use. Watch the **same** short interaction (YouTube or video clip) of a person or movie character (nonanimated) with a speech, language, hearing, or swallowing disorder at least three times. Between each viewing of the sample, note additional observation(s) on the Specified Focus Observation Form (Figure 8–3). Watch a second interaction of a different person or movie character (nonanimated) with a speech, language, hearing, or swallowing disorder at least three times. This time, complete the Open Focus Observation Form (Figure 8–4) with characteristics unspecified.

Specified Focus Observation Form

Name of client: _____ Date: _____
Purpose of observation/Questions to be answered by the observation: _____
_____

Place: _____ Individuals present: _____
Length of observation: _____
General description of procedure(s) used: _____
_____

Observer: _____

Before you begin, list characteristics you want to gather information about in the first column.

After the observation, describe examples of the behavior in columns 2 and 3. Next in column 3, form conclusions about your characteristic–would you rate it as too much, normal, or too little?

Finally summarize your observation at the bottom of the form.

Characteristic	Example	Example	Too much Normal Too Little

Summary of observation(s):

Figure 8–3. Fill out the Specified Focus Observation Form for a short interaction with a character with speech, language, hearing, or swallowing disorder.

Open Focus Observation Form

Name of client: _____ Date: _____
Purpose of observation/Questions to be answered by the observation: _____
_____

Place: _____ Individuals present: _____
Length of observation: _____
General description of procedure(s) used: _____
_____

Observer: _____

Record your observations in the space below. Summarize your findings at the bottom of the form.

Summary of observation:

Figure 8–4. Fill out the Open Focus Observation Form for a short interaction with a character with speech, language, hearing, or swallowing disorder.

Identify the strengths and limitations of both types of observation (open focus vs. specified focus).

a. Strengths of Specified Focus Observation Form:

_____
_____
_____
_____

b. Limitations Specified Focus Observation Form:

_____
_____
_____
_____

c. Strengths of Open Focus Observation Form:

d. Limitations Open Focus Observation Form:

2. Which form did you prefer? Why?

References

American Speech-Language-Hearing Association. (n.d.).Clinical standards for speech-language pathology frequently asked questions: Clinical practicum. Retrieved May 16, 2018, from https://www.asha.org/Certification/Certification-Standards-for-SLP-Clinical-Practicum/

Damico, J. S. (1988). The lack of efficacy in language therapy: A case study. *Language, Speech, and Hearing Services in Schools, 19*, 51–66.

Hall, N. (2016). Teaching observation skills: A survey of CSD practices. *Contemporary Issues in Communication Science and Disorder, 43*, 98–105.

Richards, S. B., Taylor, R. L., Ramasamy, R., & Richards, R. Y. (1999). *Single subject research*. San Diego, CA: Singular.

Simons, D. J., & Chabris, C. F. (1999), Gorillas in our midst: Sustained inattentional blindness for dynamic events. *Perception, 28*, 1059–1074.

CHAPTER 9

Synthesizing Information

Who

When synthesizing information, clinicians must be able to take the information learned from the evaluation, interpret that information accurately to make recommendations, and report that information to clients, families, and other professionals. It is not enough to complete a valid and reliable evaluation. Clinicians must take that information and translate it into something that will answer the initial question(s) and relay that information to other parties involved in a way that people without a degree in speech-language pathology or audiology can understand. Kohnert (2013) describes the process or main goals of evaluation as identifying a disorder, describing the current communication abilities, planning for treatment, and monitoring ongoing progress. Clinicians start by using all the information obtained to determine if the patient qualifies for services and if so, identify the location, type and amount of remediation recommended.

The American Speech-Language-Hearing Association (ASHA) has guidelines for clinicians in the areas of assessment (American Speech-Language-Hearing Association, n.d.). The guidelines are as follows:

The applicant for certification must have completed a program of study that included experiences sufficient in breadth and depth to achieve the following skills outcomes:

Evaluation:

- *Conduct screening and prevention procedures (including prevention activities).*
- *Collect case history information and integrate information from clients/patients, family, caregivers, teachers, and relevant others, including other professionals.*
- *Select and administer appropriate evaluation procedures, such as behavioral observations, nonstandardized and standardized tests, and instrumental procedures.*
- *Adapt evaluation procedures to meet client/patient needs.*
- *Interpret, integrate, and synthesize all information to develop diagnoses and make appropriate recommendations for intervention.*
- *Complete administrative and reporting functions necessary to support evaluation.*
- *Refer clients/patients for appropriate services.*

As you can see, not only are we doing what is best for the client by being able to synthesize assessment information, we are required to have the skills in order to be certified and practice at the highest level possible.

As clinicians, we must also remember that within our field we have many advances in the ability to diagnose disorders and plan for treatment. New technological advances help us in the identification of disorders and the implementation of therapy; however, we must not forget that test results are one piece in the puzzle. As Richard (2017) so adeptly states, "We need to remember the personal touch and importance of putting all the components together to achieve the best outcome for our clients" (p. 6).

What

Accurate and reliable evaluation information is the crucial beginning step; however, it does not stop there. A clinician must take that information along with observations, questionnaires, referral information, case history, and any other related information, and put it together to get a more complete picture of the client's communicative ability. A clinician must use all this to determine if treatment is needed, and if so, what goals and objectives will be targeted and in what order. From there, a clinician must then report the findings in terms that can be understood and be helpful to others as they try to get a better picture of the client's abilities, differences, and weaknesses.

It is important to emphasize that while standardized testing is helpful in qualifying a client for services, a clinician could miss vital information on the client's abilities if test scores are the only piece of information used. There are many examples of why additional information is needed to get a more complete idea of a client's abilities. One area that has gained more attention and research in recent years is in the assessment of bilingual clients. In a study by Ebert and Pham (2017), the authors noted that there is a heavy reliance on English standardized tests, which are not often normed with bilingual clients. Heilmann, Rojas, Iglesias, and Miller (2016) recently called language sample analysis the gold standard in language assessment with bilingual children. When information from both standardized tests and language sample analysis is synthesized, it provides a more complete picture of the client's strengths and needs.

Why

Using all information available is vital to painting the correct picture of the client's abilities. It is our responsibility as clinicians to provide the best evidence-based evaluations and treatment services. Without using all the information, a clinician could miss vital pieces or lead others to a misunderstanding of the client's ability. It is not uncommon for the standardized test results to miss the full picture of the client's abilities. A clinician must always remember that the testing done reflects that one moment in time and many variables can create a certain picture. For instance, if a child is very shy or uncomfortable in the environment, he may not respond to questions even when he has something to say. It is also possible to get test results that do not paint the entire picture. A client may be able to make sounds more clearly when saying one or two words at a time, but when talking in sentences his/her sounds become unclear and not easily understood. If a clinician takes the information from the standardized test where the client was tasked with saying one or two words at a time, it could look like the client does not have problems with articulation; but, in reality, the client cannot be understood in most instances.

As you can see, the evaluation process does not stop with formal tests, nor does your job stop with answering the question of "Does the client qualify for services?" You must also share information in a clear way that will let the client and others the client would like to share that information with know the status of their communication ability and what, if any, services are recommended.

When

Following initial evaluations, using ongoing assessment information, and at various times along the treatment path, you will need to be able to accurately synthesize information from a client. Strong clinicians are constantly assessing a client's performance to plan for treatment and should also always be updating the client and others involved of their progress and changes that need to occur to assist the client in meeting his/her goals.

Where

Synthesizing information is ongoing and thus can occur anywhere and all the time. There will be times during an evaluation and/or treatment session when you must take known information and what is happening at that moment and adjust as necessary. For instance, if an objective is written as "Client will correctly follow two-step directions with 90% accuracy over three consecutive sessions" and the client correctly follows those two-step directions every time they are given an opportunity for three consecutive sessions, you will then move to the next level such as following three-step directions.

Reporting information can also occur at any time. Perhaps you take 5 min at the end of each session to go over information with the client's family members or discuss the direction therapy is going. You will also complete daily SOAP notes, perhaps monthly or semester progress reports, and discharge reports in addition to the original evaluation report.

How

Information is typically reported in one of two ways, verbal or written, and many times a combination of both. A written report serves as a historical document for your client. Written reports can be returned to time and again to review information and specific information for your client(s). Verbal reporting is also important as this provides an easy and quick way to relay information that is pertinent to that particular moment in time. If you wanted to discuss a client's progress, it is faster to do this verbally as this information could change rapidly. For example, if you were working with a client on articulation and you wanted the family to focus on a particular sound at the beginning of words and in 2 weeks the client had moved from needing to work on that sound at the beginning of words to the end of words, it would be far more helpful to relay that information verbally as opposed to writing a report of progress and giving that to the family. You may also work on a team and during a team meeting you need to report on the progress of a client. It is more likely you report this information verbally as opposed to bringing copies of a written report for all the team members.

Regardless of the format of the presentation of information, there are several things to keep in mind:

1. You want to report accurate and clear information in the briefest way possible. This does not mean that you want to abbreviate things and shorten the report by using terms that are not common to most individuals or that you want to leave out vital information. This does, however, mean that you want to have accurate and valid information to share with others, explaining any data that you present and using terms that families and other service providers not in the field of speech pathology or audiology will understand.

2. When synthesizing information you want to look at the whole picture of the client. This means you will likely need to take the evaluation data as well as observational data and other information to get a whole picture of the client's abilities. If a client does not qualify based on standardized scores but you notice that when talking with a client they are not a successful communicator, you may need to pull other evaluation tools or use additional information such as a speech/language sample and observational information to explain how the client qualifies for services.

Top 10 Terms

Valid

Reliable

Evidence based practices

Synthesis

Observations

Questionnaires

Case history

Written report

Verbal report

Progress report

Chapter Tips

1. It is your responsibility as a clinician to use all the available information to answer the question(s) related to the client's communicative abilities.

2. You will need to be constantly evaluating how the client is doing. The evaluation does not always need to be a formal evaluation, but it is up to you to determine the appropriateness of goals/objectives and when those need to change.

3. You do not always have to give information in a written format. Most often you will be verbally discussing the progress of the client.

Activities

9-1. List information you may obtain during an evaluation session that will help determine the client's communicative ability.

_____

_____

_____

_____

9-2. Read the following scenario then determine and discuss the way(s) this particular client qualified for services.

Client is a 3 year 6 month old female. Parents report child gets frustrated often when no one understands what she is trying to say. Parents report she uses gestures, single words, and will lead you to what she wants if she cannot get it herself. She reportedly attends day care and is very interactive with other children, but also seems to experience frustration with her classmates and teachers when trying to communicate. Articulation testing reveals a standard score of 1 standard deviation below the mean. Language testing reveals scores that fall in the normal range for receptive language and 1 standard deviation below mean for expressive language. A speech sample reveals multiple sound errors in all instances when more than three words are spoken in connected speech.

_____

_____

_____

_____

9–3. Rewrite the following information in more client-friendly terminology:

Victor exhibits deficits in articulation and expressive language. These deficits are considered to be in the moderate range based on standardized scores. Services are warranted and should include caregiver training.

_____

_____

_____

_____

_____

Answers to Activities

9–1. Age, medical history, social history, observation, interview, standardized scores, speech/language sample.

9–2. This client qualifies for services based on the connected speech sample. Parent report helped to identify that the child was not being understood most of the time. Standardized scores revealed the child was below the mean in articulation and expressive language, but not at a level that typically qualifies for services (most often more than 1.5 standard deviations below the mean would be the cutoff for qualifying). The speech/language sample revealed this client had several speech sound errors during connected speech. While she did not qualify based on standardized testing, the speech/language sample revealed she was having difficulty when putting words together. Her speech sounds were no longer clear when other words were needed to relay information. You would use this information to determine treatment should begin at the phrase level versus the word level because the articulation test did not indicate problems with sound production at the word level.

9–3. Victor has communication difficulties in two different areas. The first area is articulation and indicates that Victor does not say sounds as clearly as he should for his age. He also has problems when trying to express himself or get the information he wishes to share across to the listener. Victor's communication difficulties are considered to be in the moderate range and indicate that in most circumstances he would have difficulty being understood. Speech treatment is recommended to assist him in learning to make his speech sounds more clear as well as develop language skills that would help him express his ideas, wants, and needs more effectively. Along with the individualized treatment for Victor, we will also plan to work with his friends and family members to carry over the information from clinic to home.

Wrap-Up

1. Review the ASHA skills guidelines located at the beginning of this chapter. Consider the various assessment areas and write two goals for yourself. What information or activities will you need to meet these goals (write these down as well so you can review them from time to time to see your progress)?

   Goal 1:

   _____
   _____
   _____
   _____

   Information needed:

   _____
   _____
   _____
   _____

   Activities to be completed to help reach my goal:

   _____
   _____
   _____
   _____

   Goal 2:

   _____
   _____
   _____
   _____

   Information needed:

   _____
   _____

Activities to be completed to help reach my goal:

2. Find a YouTube video of a speech/language evaluation. What standardized assessment(s) were being given? What additional information did you notice/would you use to help give you a fuller picture of the client's communicative ability? What areas would you report on and how would you report based on the information you watched in the video?

3. Think about a time when you have been given feedback based on something you did (perhaps a project for school or a report given for an evaluation you completed), what information was most helpful for you? What information do you wish you had been given? Were you given the opportunity to ask questions after receiving the feedback? Did you ask for clarification? Use this situation to help guide you through the process of gathering information, synthesizing the information, and reporting on the information.

References

American Speech-Language-Hearing Association (n.d.) 2014 ASHA certification standards in speech-language pathology. Retrieved October 24, 2017, from https://www.asha.org/Certification/2014-Speech-Language-Pathology-Certification-Standards/#Standard_VI

Ebert, K. D., & Pham, G. (2017). Synthesiznig information from language samples and standardized tests in school-age bilingual assessment. *Language, Speech, and Hearing Services in Schools, 48*, 42–55.

Heilmann, J. J., Rojas, R., Iglesias, A., & Miller, J. F. (2016). Clinical impact of wordless picture storybooks on bilingual narrative language production: A comparison of the "frog" stories. *International Journal of Language & Communication Disorders, 43*, 191–204.

Kohnert, K. (2013). *Language disorders in bilingual children and adults* (2nd ed.) San Diego, CA: Plural.

Richard, G. L. (2017). The "big picture" diagnostician. *The ASHA Leader, 22*(2), 6–7.

CHAPTER 10

Report Writing

Who

Every clinician is responsible for writing appropriate assessment reports (Pannbacker, Middleton, Vekovius, & Sanders, 2001). These include the initial assessment/diagnostic report (before treatment is begun), ongoing assessment notes (SOAP notes), progress reports or reevaluation reports (after the client has been enrolled in remediation services for a period of time), and dismissal or final reports (at the end of the remediation process). This written information is read by clients, families, funding agencies, and other professionals. Reports are your opportunity to provide a clear, concise, and permanent record of the information you have gathered. A report needs to be detailed and concise at the same time. Obtaining insurance payment for your services is reliant on your ability to provide required information within your reports. What you select to include or not include, the way you organize and state the information, the data and explanations you provide, and the clearness of your supported conclusions and recommendations are all of vital importance. It is sad but true that a clinician can be the best diagnostician in the world, but unless he/she can communicate information in a written format, he/she is doing the client a disservice. Thankfully, clinical writing can be taught through means such as observation and exposure to authentic clinical writing (Hull, 2013) and specifically teaching the "genre" of record writing (Oglensky & Davidson, 2009).

What

A written report is a summary of the relevant information about the client's speech, language, and hearing characteristics. Most reports contain aspects of relevant past information, current level of functioning, and future recommendations. This section of the chapter will emphasize the initial diagnostic assessment report. Later in the chapter, the initial report will be compared to ongoing notes and the progress report will be compared to the final report.

The initial diagnostic report documents the evaluation performed to identify the type and severity of speech, language, or hearing disorder and recommendations for enrollment/nonenrollment and/or referral. To aid in clarity of information, headings are employed to separate the report into content sections. Typical sections of a report are as follows.

The first section in a diagnostic report provides the **Identifying Information**. The accuracy of this information is critical. Always have the client or an informant confirm the accuracy of this identifying information at the start of the assessment. The name of the site or facility where the assessment was performed is usually centered on the top of the page. Identifying information including the client's name, address, phone number, birthdate, file number, diagnosis, date of evaluation, and clinician's name are presented in a list format. A specific site may require additional information such as parents' names, school status, age, referral source, or clinician's provider number. This first section is presented in a list format, while the remaining sections of the report are written primarily in paragraph form.

The next section provides a restatement of the identifying information and the reason for the referral. This paragraph typically contains the client's first and last name, age, gender, name of evaluation site, date of evaluation, person who referred the client, and reason for the referral. An example paragraph under the heading **Reason for Referral** would state: "Jersey Jones, a 6-year-10-month-old female, was referred to the University Speech and Hearing Clinic on February 15, 2018, by her doctor, John C. Hener. A high occurrence of dysfluencies was the reason for the referral."

The third section, **History**, may be separated into subheadings such as prenatal and birth history, developmental history, medical history, social history, educational history, work history, and so forth. The clinician determines what information from this particular client's past is relevant to the questions being addressed and whether subheadings are needed to facilitate the organization of this information. An example of history information would state: "Mrs. Edwards reported that Tom was difficult to understand by individuals not familiar with his speech pattern. Developmental milestones were obtained at the appropriate times. Numerous ear infections occurred between the ages of 5 months and 4 years and were treated with antibiotics. Pressure equalizing tubes were inserted at the age of 4 years."

The fourth section, **Assessment Information (Findings or Results)**, may be separated into subheadings such as observations, oral peripheral, articulation, language comprehension and production, voice, fluency, swallowing, literacy, hearing, memory, and so forth. The selection of specific subheadings and the order of the headings will differ depending on the individualized assessments given. When describing the results from a standardized test, the name of the test is given in italics and a brief description of the area(s) the test addresses is provided. The results are stated and an interpretation of what these results indicate is provided. An example paragraph under the subheading, articulation would state: "Donald's articulation skills were assessed utilizing the *Goldman-Fristoe 3 Test of Articulation (GFTA-3)*. The *GFTA-3* is a norm-referenced instrument designed to assess articulation of the consonant sounds in standard American English for individuals aged 2 through 21. The *GFTA-3* has a mean of 100 and a standard deviation of +/−15. This means that standard scores between 85 and 115 are considered within the average range. Donald presented with a speech sound score of 95, which indicated that his articulation ability was within the average range for his age group." Test scores are augmented with details of observed strengths and weaknesses as well as unique findings. In Donald's example, the paragraph would continue by stating: "Errors were noted in /l/ blend words where the /l/ was omitted from the blend. The word "blue" was produced as "bue." The sound in word errors were also noted in conversational speech. Since Donald was 7 years and 4 months, his GFTA-3 standard score, if only /l/ blends were in error, was 95 and his percentile rank was 37." Following the assessment results, a **Summary and Recommendations** section is provided (sometimes these are reported as two separate sections). This section integrates all the results from the individual sections. It includes consideration of both subjective (e.g., impressions and observations) and objective information (e.g., test results and data). In the summary portion, a classification of the disorder, severity level, and prognosis (a consideration of factors that influence the likelihood that the client will benefit from treatment) are included. An example of a summary for a patient following a stroke might state: "Mr. Hamilton demonstrated severe deficits in all receptive and expressive language areas. This is consistent with the diagnosis of global aphasia. Enrollment in speech and language remediation is recommended for 4 days a week for 50 min to address comprehension and functional communication needs prior to medical discharge. Prognosis appears guarded based on the patient's motivation and family involvement." The recommendations portion should be as specific as possible. When remediation is recommended, the frequency (how many times a week) and intensity (length of time) of the treatment should be described. A set of goals should be provided and the current level of functioning specified for each goal. Often, this is a percentage, frequency measure, or time period obtained on a baseline measure. When the recommendations include a referral, the reason for the referral should be stated. An example of a continuation of the summary and recommendations for Mr. Hamilton might state: "The goals for Mr. Hamilton should include: (1) to express five wants/needs within the 50 min session time using speech, gestures, or pictures (current level is one want/need expressed); (2) to make a choice between two items within a functional task such as eating, dressing, or listening to music (current level is 0/5 trials); and (3) to engage with family members for a 15 min period of time (current level is 5 min)." While it is ideal to determine functioning level for each goal before the end of the diagnostic session, if baseline information was unable to be determined by the end of the diagnostic session, it should be the first procedure completed in the initial treatment session.

Finally, all reports must contain a **Signature**. The clinician signs above his/her typed name, degree, and professional certification. An example signature line for a clinician would be, "Mary Smith, MA, CCC, SLP."

Why

Reports are written to document and disseminate information across interested parties. In practice, reports are necessary to secure funding for services. The types of previously mentioned reports differ in their purposes and this in turn leads to differences in their characteristics. The charts provided in this section compare the initial diagnostic report to the ongoing SOAP note and the progress report to the final report.

At one level, SOAP notes represent "mini-assessment" reports. SOAP stands for subjective (S), objective (O), assessment (A), and plan (P), and are written to document the daily treatment session (for additional information and practice writing session notes see Hambrecht & Rice, 2011). Table 10–1 presents a comparison between an initial diagnostic report and a SOAP note, and highlights the similarities and differences between the two written documents.

Table 10–1. Comparison between Initial Diagnostic Report and SOAP Note

Characteristic	Initial Diagnostic Report	SOAP Note
Purpose	To identify the type and severity of speech, language, or hearing disorders and recommend enrollment/nonenrollment and/or referral.	To track therapy progress and recommend steps for next session.
Frequency	Written prior to enrollment.	Written daily.
Headings	Identifying information, history, assessment results, summary, recommendations, and signature.	Subjective, objective, assessment, plan, and signature.
Relevant past information	History may include medical, developmental, social, and educational.	S might include a report from a parent or teacher concerning incidents prior to the therapy session.
Current level of functioning	Critical component presented as subjective and objective information. Sections of the report include assessment results, observations, and summary.	Primarily reported in the O section as percentages, frequency, or rate data gathered in the session. Can be reported in the S section as observations or impressions.
Future recommendations	Prognosis and recommendation sections of report.	P describes the plan for future session(s).
Length	Will vary but approximately 3 to 5 pages.	Will vary but approximately half to 1 page.

A progress report typically emphasizes the change in performance from the initial or last progress report to the level of performance at the end of the current treatment period. The final report is, in fact, the last or final progress report where discharge is recommended. Table 10–2 compares the progress and final reports on the same characteristics previously used to compare the initial diagnostic report and the SOAP note.

Table 10–2. Comparison of a Progress Report and a Final Report

Characteristic	Progress Report	Final Report
Purpose	To identify the changes that have occurred due to therapy from the initial enrollment or the last progress report and recommend specific next steps. Were goals met and what additional goals need to be addressed?	To identify the changes that have occurred due to therapy from the initial enrollment or the last progress report and recommend discharge of patient. Status of goals.
Frequency	Written periodically during the therapy process. How frequently will depend on the site.	Written once prior to discharge.
Headings	Identifying information including diagnosis, start date, and frequency of treatment sessions; goals and objectives; level of functioning for each objective at beginning of treatment period and end of treatment period; recommendations; and signature.	Identifying information including diagnosis, start date, and frequency of treatment sessions; goals and objectives; level of functioning for each objective at beginning of treatment period and end of treatment period; recommendations for follow up; and signature.
Relevant past information	Level of functioning at the beginning of treatment period.	Level of functioning at the beginning of treatment period.
Current level of functioning	Level of function at end of treatment period including current level of functioning for any new goals/objectives.	Level of function at end of treatment period.
Future recommendations	Recommendation for change(s) to treatment plan.	Recommendation for discharge and follow-up session.
Length	Will vary, but approximately 1 page.	Will vary, but approximately 1 page.

When

Reports need to be completed in a timely fashion. They should be written as soon as possible after the completion of the evaluation (in the case of the initial diagnostic report), the session (in the case of the SOAP note), the prescribed evaluation period (in the case of the progress report), or the remediation services (in the case of the final report). Work sites will typically have a specified turnaround time for reports.

Where

Reports are confidential and should be maintained in secure files whether in a paper format or an electronic format. A site will maintain the documentation for at least five years.

How

A student doing an internship placement suggested a process to improve efficiency and professional writing as she learned to write more confidently at a new placement site (B. Branch, personal communication, March 29, 2016). Branch suggested creating a type of terminology glossary, an organized listing of phrases that could be used or modified while documenting client behavior in reports or session notes. Her list included such items as "Patient was alert, pleasant, and happily reported having had her first cup of coffee this morning since admission" for an *S* entry in a SOAP note. Her list also included phrases such as "Patient was reclined in bed with wife present for evaluation. Oral mechanism exam revealed labial, lingual, and buccal weakness; apraxic-like impairment with facial exercises (raising/lowering eyebrows); and difficulty with labial retraction/protrusion requiring maximum cues and assistance." Also noted was "lingual deviation to right side" for an *O* entry in a SOAP note. Worthington and Fleck (2012) provided a list of words to avoid and a list of words to use in a report. Words they suggested to be avoided included "struggled," "suffered," "dealing with," "succumb," "sadly," "devastated," "working on," "isn't/can't" (all contractions), and "did therapy with." Words to use included "exhibited difficulty," "displayed/demonstrated," "assessed/evaluated," "treated/remediated," "provided," "established," and "implemented."

Report writing is different from creative writing in that there are many instances where similar sentences will appear across reports. This is especially true when results are within the normal range. Examples include "An oral facial examination revealed normal structure and function of the oral mechanism." and "A pure tone hearing screening revealed hearing within normal limits bilaterally." While report writing is different from creative writing, this does not mean you do not follow the rules of grammar, punctuation, and formatting learned from past writing instruction. Use spell and grammar check and the thesaurus function on your computer to your advantage. Always proofread your written work for form and truthfulness of the information provided.

Reports are often written in past tense as you are reporting on procedures and observations that have been completed. Mentally inserting the phrase "at the time of the evaluation" before the sentence can help in the use of past tense writing in reports. Check your specific work site for the preferred tense. "I," "me," and "my" are not commonly used in reports. Typically, "The clinician noted" would be used instead of "I noted." Also remember to use person first language, placing the person before the disability. Thus, state the "individual with dysarthria" instead of the "dysarthric individual." Similarly, the client does not belong to the clinician; thus, "the client" would be utilized instead of "my client" or "his/her client."

This chapter has contained numerous "rules" to help you when writing reports. The following is a summary list of the suggestions presented:

- Complete the paperwork required in a timely fashion
- Maintain the confidentiality of all reports
- Avoid negatively charged or biased terms
- Avoid contractions and overused words
- Use well-worded "pat phrases or sentences" when appropriate
- Follow the rules of grammar, punctuation, and formatting
- Proof for form and content prior to signing
- Use past tense
- Refer to yourself as "the clinician" instead of "I"
- Value the person by using person first language and avoiding "my client" or "her/his client"

Top 10 Terms

Confidentiality

Identifying information

Initial assessment report

Person first language

Professional appearance

Progress report

Prognosis

Signature line

SOAP note

Final report

Chapter Tips

1. Always find samples of reports from your organization or place of employment. This will provide you with the "model" from which to format your report. Matching the sample is a good rule of thumb to follow when starting at a new

placement or work site. Check with your site to see if templates of reports are available.

2. Reports afford you an opportunity to present your "professional appearance" to numerous constituents, some of whom may never meet you in person. Do not underestimate the importance of your written "professional appearance." Errors in grammar, word selection, or typos will call into question your level of knowledge or expertise. Attention to detail and accuracy are essential in reports, so always proof your reports and read them carefully before signing. Never sign any report without having read it thoroughly. When you sign a report, you are attesting to its accuracy.

Activities

10–1. Decide if each statement best describes the initial diagnostic report (IDR), the session notes (SOAP), the progress report (PR), or the final report (FR). Place the correct initials IDR, SOAP, PR, or FR before each statement.

1. _____ Discharges the patient from services
2. _____ Written daily
3. _____ Documents goal outcome for a specified time period
4. _____ Likely to be the longest of the 4 reports
5. _____ Identifies the initial diagnosis and severity level
6. _____ Includes a detailed history section

10–2. Rewrite each sentence by replacing the italicized word or words with a better word choice. Next, add a meaningful additional sentence that could follow the provided sentence.

1. The client *struggled* with the sentence completion task.

   _____

   _____

2. Mr. Jones *suffered* his first stroke on May 1, 2017.

   _____

   _____

3. *I did therapy with* Mary for a semester beginning on September 6, 2018.

   _____

   _____

Chapter 10 • Report Writing 99

4. Mr. and Mrs. Smith were *devastated* when they were informed by the doctor that their daughter, Sue, was born with Down syndrome two days after her birth.

5. The patient *isn't demonstrating* difficulties during feeding.

6. *Me and Tommy* reviewed last semester's vocabulary words at the start of the session to establish baseline.

7. *Mr. Perry's effect* during the session remained flat.

8. The group session consisted of *tree aphasic clients* and their caregivers.

9. *Regardless of the cues presented, I was unable to illicit* a correct /k/ production.

10. On June 5, 2018, Andrew First, a 7-year-old male, is being referred to the Speech and Hearing Center by Dr. k. Truly, a pediatrician.

Answers to Activities

10–1

1. FR
2. SOAP
3. PR
4. IDR
5. IDR
6. IDR

10–2

1. The client demonstrated difficulty with the sentence completion task. He correctly completed 2/10 items without prompts.
2. Mr. Jones had his initial stroke on May 1, 2017. Review of his medical file revealed no speech, language, or swallowing difficulties as a result of the initial stoke.
3. Mary was enrolled in therapy for a semester beginning on September 6, 2018. At the time of enrollment, Mary produced /s/ in the initial position of words with 10% accuracy.
4. Mr. and Mrs. Smith were informed by the doctor that their daughter, Sue, was born with Down syndrome two days after her birth. Sue was born prematurely at 28 weeks gestation.
5. The patient did not demonstrate difficulties during feeding. Continuation of a modified diet of solids and nectar-thick liquids was recommended.
6. Tommy reviewed last semester's vocabulary words at the start of the session to establish a baseline. He correctly defined 70% (14/20) of the terms using grammatically correct sentences.
7. Mr. Perry's affect during the session remained flat. Modeling and instruction on word emphasis within a sentence was ineffective (0/10 correct).
8. The group session consisted of three clients with aphasia and their caregivers. The interaction centered on availability of support services within the community.
9. Regardless of the cues presented, the clinician was unable to elicit a correct /k/ production. The phonemes on which the client was stimulable will be targeted first.
10. On June 5, 2018, Andrew First, a 7-year-old male, was referred to the Speech and Hearing Center by Dr. K. Truly, a pediatrician. Andrew's delayed speech and language development were the reasons for the referral.

Wrap-Up

1. Write five phrases or sentences that you might use to start your own glossary for professional writing.

    1. _____
    2. _____
    3. _____
    4. _____
    5. _____

2. How can a report be both detailed and concise at the same time?

    _____
    _____
    _____
    _____

3. Identify six pieces of information that are common in the first paragraph of an initial diagnostic report.

    1. _____
    2. _____
    3. _____
    4. _____
    5. _____
    6. _____

4. Every writer has areas of strengths and limitations. Identify your personal strengths and limitations as a report writer. Next, identify a plan of how you can begin to address one of your limitations.

    My strengths are:

    _____
    _____
    _____
    _____

My limitations are:

_____
_____
_____
_____

One way to begin to address the limitation listed previously:

_____
_____
_____
_____

5. One set of terms that can give an inexperienced writer difficulties are homonyms: words that sound the same but differ in spelling and meaning. Spell check does not catch these errors so you need to be vigilant. Write a definition for each term.

- buy

  _____

- by

  _____

- whether

  _____

- weather

  _____

- to

  _____

- too

  _____

- two

  _____

- cite

- site

- pale

- pail

- there

- their

6. Compose a list of five prognostic indicators that would be perceived as positive and five that would be perceived as negative. Enter this into Table 10–3.

Table 10–3. List of Positive and Negative Prognostic Indicators

#	Positive Prognostic Indicators	Negative Prognostic Indicators
1		
2		
3		
4		
5		

7. Write a signature line you will use following your completion of a master's degree and obtaining your Certification of Clinical Competence (CCC) from the American Speech-Language-Hearing Association (ASHA).

References

Goldman, R., & Fristoe, M. (2015). Goldman-Fristoe Test of Articulation (3rd ed., GFTA-3) [Assessment instrument]. Austin, TX: Pro-Ed.

Hambrecht, G., & Rice, T. (2011). *Clinical observation a guide for students in speech, language, and hearing.* Sudbury, MA: Jones & Bartlett Learning.

Hull, M. (2013). Learning and teaching clinical writing. *The European Medical Writers Association, 22*(1), 29–33. doi: 10.1179/2047480612Z.00000000083

Oglensky, B. D., & Davidson, E. J. (2009). Teaching and learning through clinical report-writing genres. *The International Journal of Learning, 16,* 139–152.

Pannbacker, M., Middleton, G., Vekovius, G. T., & Sanders, K. L. (2001) Report writing for speech-language pathologist and audiologists. Austin, TX: Pro-Ed.

Worthington, T., & Fleck, C. (2012). *Therapy notes & writing guidelines for students.* Poster session presented at the American Speech-Language-Hearing Association Convention, Atlanta, GA.

CHAPTER 11

Ongoing Assessment

Who

Ongoing data is collected on every client on your case load throughout the remediation process. The extent, type, and frequency of the data collected will vary depending on the specific needs of the individual client and his/her goals and objectives. Just as treatment is individualized for a given client, so too is ongoing data collection. The clinician is also not the only person responsible for the collection of data. Family members, friends, teachers, aids, and other staff all have the potential to serve as data collectors. They each bring a valuable and unique focus to the ongoing assessment process. Therapy, either directly or indirectly, involves those others who can participate in ongoing data collection by describing current events that impacted the client, participating in practice opportunities, reporting on goal progress/attainment outside of therapy, and/or providing satisfaction information. Capturing the information from these informed others is important to ensure that therapy is relevant and that changes are not limited to the therapy room or the therapist as the conversational partner. Finally, the clients themselves are important data accumulators. Client reports, frequency counts, examples, perceptions, and reflections all inform the ongoing assessment process.

What

Ongoing data differs from the initial data used to support enrollment of a client, progress data used to document benchmarks or milestones in the therapy process, and final data used to support dismissal recommendations. Ongoing data has a more formative assessment purpose, while the initial, progress, or final data serve a more summative assessment function. Formative assessment informs the teaching/learning process so adjustments can be made to improve the learning process and has been found to enhance retention and application of information by the learner (Persellin & Daniels, 2014). Formative assessment is usually reported in a session note termed a SOAP note. The SOAP note format (Subjective, Objective, Assessment, and Plan) allows for an organized presentation of daily session information (Golper, 2010).

The subjective information reported often includes impressions or observations made by the clinician or reported to the clinician by staff, family members, or the client. Information passed on by others that is not recorded in the notes fails to become part of the permanent record and thus can easily be overlooked. What the clinician notes in the S portion can also influence and explain the A and P portions of the process.

The objective information reported can include a variety of data reflecting the progress toward the client's goals. There are common types of objective measurements used to report ongoing data in the field of speech-language pathology and audiology (Richards, Taylor, Ramasamy, & Richards, 1999). Several of these are identified, briefly described, and presented as an example within a SOAP note (an O statement) in the following text:

- Percentages:
  Percentages are a very common form of data. The number of correct responses are divided by the total number of opportunities and the result is multiplied by 100. Accompanying this percentage may be the fraction form of the number correct/opportunities in parenthesis (e.g., 1/2, 5/10, or 50/100). Knowing the number of opportunities in addition to the percentage, while at some level redundant, can influence the confidence the reader has in the representativeness or clear pattern reflected in the results. Typically, whole numbers are reported for data in percentages. O: Betty produced the initial /r/ in words with 70% accuracy (14/20), in sentences with 30% accuracy (4/12), and in conversation with 1% accuracy (1/16).

- Frequency counts:
  Frequency is the number of responses that occur in a time period. Totaling the tallied occurrence of a behavior is a frequency measure. The period of time and type of activity that occurs in the time period should be kept consistent to facilitate the comparison of frequency counts over time. O: Joe spontaneously utilized a question word three times in a 5-min conversation during a topic card description task.

- Rate:
  Rate is an appropriate measure when the time period being evaluated varies (unlike frequency counts where the time period is held constant). Rate is determined by number of responses divided by the number of minutes. Session notes may include a combination of measurement types. O: Andrew demonstrated a rate of speech of 220 words per minute during connected speech. His dysfluency index was 40%.

- Duration:
  Duration is the length of time it takes for a behavior to occur from start to finish. Duration measures can be used for a wide variety of focus behaviors including length of a tantrum, response time (length of time from question being asked until response is begun), length of a sustained /s/, or length of a dysfluent block. O: Fred remained engaged at the table task for 5 min and 30 sec before throwing the items on the floor.

- Instrumentation measures:
  With the advent of new technology, measures of fundamental characteristics of voice and swallowing are readily available. When instrumentation is used, the clinician needs to make sure the equipment is regularly calibrated (checked for accuracy of output). O: Mr. Anderson's pitch, while counting from 1 to 20, was 166 Hz at the start of today's session and 162 at the end of the session. Pitch breaks decreased as humming exercises were practiced.

The assessment portion of the SOAP note brings the S and O data together to describe changes from prior sessions, identify effectiveness of cues or techniques, and, in general, explain the impact of the data on therapy materials and procedures. The beginning clinician needs to take care to evaluate the data provided in S and O and not merely restate the information.

The plan sets the stage for future sessions. Bearing in mind the assessment of the subjective and objective information just presented, the clinician now utilizes this information to identify what should be changed and what should remain unchanged to enhance client learning. This could include modifications to materials, procedures, communication partners, room setup, cueing system, target words, level of support, and order of objectives addressed—just to name a few of the possible modifications a clinician could plan.

Why

There are numerous reasons why ongoing assessment occurs. These reasons include documenting progress, checking to see if it is time to change or modify goals/objectives, determining if the treatment and not some extraneous variable/treatment (such as a medical treatment/procedure or an educational opportunity/experience) is responsible for a behavior change, passing on information to future clinicians, encouraging client's retention and application of material learned, and maintaining legal documentation. Funding through Medicaid, Medicare, or private insurance for services requires reports of data-driven practices.

Olswang and Bain (1994) identified four clinical question addressed using ongoing data:

"Is the child responding to the treatment program?"

"Is significant and important change occurring?"

"Is treatment responsible for the change?"

"How long should a therapy target be treated?" (p. 55)

The data they used to address the questions took a variety of forms. Three of the forms of data regularly collected in the field of speech-language pathology and audiology include therapy task responses, probes, and informant reports. The following text further describes these three general forms of data generation.

- Therapy task responses or treatment responses are gathered in the therapy session as the client applies the strategies and techniques being trained. Level of cueing or support as well as difficulty of task (i.e., word level or spontaneous speech) are included when relevant.

- Probes or trial items are gathered to investigate generalization of target behavior(s) to nontrained targets, new partners, or nontrained environment/situations. The probe scoring system (Hall, Adams, Hesketh, & Nightingale, 1998) was developed specifically to document small but significant changes in speech production for children with severe speech disorders. Probing may also occur to aid in selection of targets appropriate for the next therapy session(s) (Hodson & Paden, 1991). Former baseline data that is now reoccurring tracks change from the initial baseline and is a type of probe data. While no one probe list is representative of all probe lists, a probe list for an articulation disorder is provided in the following numbered list as an example.

If Loraine, a 7-year-old female, had a goal of production of /s/ and /z/ in the final position of words with 80% accuracy given a picture stimulus, the probe list might include the following items. Note that only the /s/ (not the /z/) is currently targeted in therapy and none of the items on the list were training target words (these words were used only to assess generalization of learning). A rationale as to why each item was selected is provided in parenthesis following the item.

1. "Sis" (a simple palindrome where the initial /s/ may facilitate the final /s/ production)
2. "Mice" (single syllable word)
3. "Mouse" (single syllable word with a different vowel)
4. "Geese" (single syllable word with a different vowel)
5. "Fireplace" (two syllable word may increase the difficulty level)
6. "Asparagus" (four syllable word may increase the difficulty level)
7. "Hats" (single syllable word with a /ts/ blend, placement for /t/ may facilitate the /s/ production)
8. "Posts" (single syllable with a /sts/ may increase the difficulty level)
9. "Months" (single syllable word with a voiceless "th" before the /s/ may increase the difficulty level)
10. "A white house and two black houses" (multiple /s/ words in a phrase may increase the difficulty level)
11. "Six trucks" (multiple /s/ including a /ks/ may increase the difficulty level)
12. "Eyes" (looking for cognate pair generalization to a final /z/ word)
13. "Nose" (looking for cognate pair generalization to a final /z/ word)
14. "Pans" (looking for cognate pair generalization to a final /z/ word)
15. "Clothes" (looking for cognate pair generalization to a final /z/ word)
16. "Six drums" (looking for cognate pair generalization to a final /z/ word and final /s/ in same item may increase the difficulty level)

A probe list such as the one above would be presented periodically, perhaps every two or three weeks, to track in-session generalization changes over time. The clinician might predict that the child would show gradual improvement by correctly producing items in a progressive order from 1 to 15, but children surprise us all the time and learn differently than our expectations. That is precisely why we track individual data.

Generalization probing across partners and situations involves tracking the client's goals while he/she is interacting with a variety of people in a variety of situations. The clinician can observe the client in social situations; at home, work, or school; or even on the phone, either in person or through taped recordings. Generalization probes should be conducted throughout the therapy process and not merely when dismissal is anticipated.

Informant reports document solicited input from relevant stakeholders including family, staff, and the client. When soliciting input from others on the client's progress, information should be solicited in an open-ended, nonleading fashion. A question such as, "Tell me about any changes you have heard in Mr. Sanchez's speech in the last week" is less leading than, "Mr. Sanchez is talking so much louder since he has been in therapy, isn't he?" The client's views on progress should also be included when soliciting informant reports.

When

There is a balance between time spent collecting ongoing data and time spent delivering treatment. Beginning clinicians often struggle to establish a good balance by either forgetting to collect consistent regular data or by spending an excessive amount of time collecting data to the detriment of teaching time. To maximize the teaching time, data collection needs to be streamlined.

Data record sheets with the client's name, file number, date, and time can help with the organization of the information being obtained as well as the maintenance of the information over time. Data record sheets can be as specific (pertinent to this particular client and his/her goals) or as open-ended (adaptable to a variety of clients and goals) as the clinician deems necessary. Some clinicians record a therapy group on a single sheet, while others prefer a different score sheet for each client. The variety of data collection sheets is vast, but all capture the information so it can be summarized in the session notes.

Where

To be externally valid, data collection needs to occur across settings and communication partners. Data collected outside of therapy also promotes awareness that changes in speech and language need to be generalized beyond the therapy setting. Therapy task responses and in-session probing occur in the therapy setting, while across setting generalization probes and informant reports are collected in settings outside the therapy situation.

How

The techniques used to collect ongoing data will vary across clients. The actual data form (i.e., specific or open-ended) used for collection and type of data collected (i.e., percentages, frequency counts, rate, duration or instrumentation measurements) is a clinical decision made to best monitor the individual client's treatment progress. While data collection needs to occur regularly, this does not mean data on every minute of the therapy session must be kept. A balance between assessing time and teaching time is vital. The clinician needs to collect sufficient data to provide formative feedback and to document therapy progress within and beyond the therapy session, while at the same time providing appropriate remediation.

Top 10 Terms

Calibrated

Duration

Frequency counts

Formative assessment

Instrumentation measures

Percentages

Probes

Rate

SOAP note

Summative assessment

Chapter Tips

1. Write your SOAP note documenting your ongoing data as soon after your session as possible. Delaying can result in increased inaccuracies. It is also important to do your billing paperwork in a timely fashion.

2. Accurate and complete documentation records are a clinician's best defense when litigation or due process hearings occur. Maintain neat, organized records in a secure location.

3. The SOAP note is focused on what the client did and not what the clinician did. You would write, "The client produced" and not "The clinician presented."

Activities

11–1. Match the information described to the type of data it represents. Use P for percentage, F for frequency count, R for rate, D for duration, and I for instrumentation measure.

1. Number of words spoken every session.
2. Number of intelligible words out of total number of words spoken.

3. Number of words named in 2 min.
4. Time it takes to name 10 animals.
5. All the animals the child can recall.
6. Pitch measured on the Visi-Pitch III.
7. Number of words the client judges to be at an appropriate pitch out of number of words attempted.
8. Number of words the teacher aid identifies as having a "good /r/" while reading a paragraph aloud compared to number of /r/ words in the paragraph.
9. Length of a stuttering block in a conversational sample.
10. Number of blocks in a conversational sample.

11–2. Match the information described to the form of data generated. Use TTR for therapy task response, IP for in-session probe, PSP for new partner or situation probe, IRO for informant report by others, and IRC for informant report by client.

1. Clinician going into the classroom and recording the percentage of correct /r/ sounds used in a reading aloud task.
2. Teacher reporting on her perception of the client's articulation while retelling a story book he made in therapy the day before.
3. Client describing his homework assignment of using his fluency techniques while making three phone calls to various businesses and asking for hours of operation.
4. After discussing and practicing topic maintenance, recording the last 5 min of a therapy conversation and tracking the number of inappropriate topic changes.
5. Having child say one of his consonants in error with the vowels /i/, /a/, and /u/ in the initial, medial, and final positions (i.e., /if/, /ifi/, /fi/) at the start of the session. One consonant a day is recorded until all eight error consonants are surveyed.

Answers to Activities

11–1

1. F
2. P
3. R
4. D
5. F

6. I
7. P
8. P
9. DF

11–2

1. PSP
2. IRO
3. IRC
4. TTR
5. IP

Wrap-Up

1. Describe a specific formative assessment example and a specific summative assessment example you have taken in your college career.

   Formative assessment example =

   _____
   _____

   Summative assessment example =

   _____
   _____

2. Identify three specific medical treatments/procedures and three educational opportunities/experiences that could result in a significant gain in a child or adult with a speech, language, hearing, or swallowing disorder.

   Medical treatments/procedures =

   1. _____
   2. _____
   3. _____

   Educational opportunities/experiences =

   1. _____
   2. _____
   3. _____

Chapter 11 • Ongoing Assessment   113

3. Develop a data collection sheet for keeping track of the probe list data for Loraine (presented in the Why portion of this chapter). Do not forget to include important identifying information.

   Data collection sheet:

   _____
   _____
   _____
   _____

   Give a rationale for your probe data collection sheet format.

   _____
   _____
   _____
   _____

   Would you consider your data sheet to be specific or more open ended?

   _____
   _____
   _____
   _____

4. Philip is a 20-year-old college student with a moderate fluency disorder. Describe a possible therapy task response, in-session probe, new partner or situation probe, informant report by others, and informant report by client.

   Therapy task response =

   _____
   _____

   In-session probe =

   _____
   _____

   New partner or situation probe =

   _____
   _____

Informant report by others =

Informant report by client =

5. The authors note that, "There is a balance between time spent collecting ongoing data and time spent in delivering treatment." Ideally, how much time of a 30-min session do you think should be devoted to data collection and how much to delivering the treatment? Find a classmate, more advanced student, and/or SLP and talk about this issue. Present your recommendation for time division.

References

Golper, L. A. C. (2010). *Medical speech-language pathology: A desk reference* (3rd ed.). Clifton Park, NY: Delmar Cengage.

Hall, R., Adams. C., Hesketh, A., & Nightingale, K. (1998). The measurement of intervention effects in developmental phonological disorders. *International Journal of Language & Communication Disorders, 33*(Suppl.), 445–450.

Hodson, B. W., & Paden, E. P. (1991). *Targeting intelligible speech* (2nd ed.). Austin, TX: Pro Ed.

Olswang, L. B., & Bain, B. (1994, September). Data collection: Monitoring children's treatment progress. *American Journal of Speech Language Pathology, 3(3)*, 55–66.

Persellin, D. C., & Daniels, M. B. (2014). *A concise guide to improving student learning*. Sterling, VI: Stylus.

Richards, S. B., Taylor, R. L., Ramasamy, R., & Richards, R. Y. (1999). *Single subject research applications in educational and clinical settings*. San Diego, CA: Singular.

CHAPTER 12

Hearing Assessment

Who

As you know, hearing problems can lead to speech/language problems. Prior to testing for speech/language difficulties, the clinician must make sure they know the status of the client's hearing abilities. If the client has had a recent audiogram or hearing screening, the clinician may not need to rescreen the client; however, best practice would be to verify that the client is hearing at a level that is adequate for testing on that particular day.

What

Hearing loss at any age can result in problems with a person's speech/language abilities. For young children, hearing loss can cause problems with hearing sounds clearly; thus, leading to them not being able to say the sounds clearly. Adults who have significant difficulty hearing can also experience problems making their sounds clearly because they cannot monitor their voice as well. This can happen even if the adult had normal or near-normal hearing until they developed the significant hearing loss. At any age, a hearing loss can cause problems with being able to monitor your own speech production, so speech sounds may not be as clear.

On the language side, a client who has hearing loss may have problems hearing well enough to develop vocabulary, pragmatic information, the ability to follow multistep directions, among others. Hearing loss of any type or degree that occurs in infancy or childhood, can cause problems with the development of a child's spoken language, reading and/or writing skills, as well as academic performance (Madell & Flexer, 2014). For adults who develop hearing loss, we expect to see more problems with receptive language, pragmatics, and cognition. If a person is not hearing well, they often express problems with being able to follow conversations, which often lead to feelings of isolation and less involvement in social situations. Repeated difficulty leads to more isolation, which leads to less interactions with others and declines in cognition. A study conducted by Lin et al. (2011) revealed that adults with mild hearing loss are twice as likely to develop dementia as those with normal hearing, and as the hearing loss increased, the level of developing dementia also increased.

Determining if a person has hearing that is adequate for speech/language testing is vital to making sure the results you get are valid and reliable. If a person has a hearing loss and you do not know that before testing, you could end up with test results that are not an accurate reflection of that person's communicative ability because he/she may have been struggling to hear the directions or questions for test items.

Why

Hearing loss can occur due to a variety of factors. A conductive hearing loss is typically medically or surgically treatable as this is a problem that occurs in the outer or middle part of the ear. A conductive loss can range from a slight hearing loss to a moderately-severe hearing loss. A person with a moderately-severe hearing loss would struggle to hear someone talking at normal conversation levels. Causes of conductive hearing loss range from impacted cerumen (wax in the ear), to fluid in the middle ear, to otosclerosis (where the stapes, or last bone of the middle ear, gets fixated in the oval window and sound cannot be transmitted easily to the inner ear). Some conductive problems come and go quickly, such as an ear infection that temporarily causes problems with hearing, while some conductive problems continue over time and often get worse as time progresses, such as otosclerosis. If a client were to have a conductive hearing loss on the day of testing, they may not report long-term hearing problems but may still have difficulty hearing clearly, hearing soft speech, or hearing in the presence of background noise. Any of these could easily skew the results of your test.

A sensorineural hearing loss is a problem typically in the inner ear or beyond and is not medically or surgically treatable. Cochlear implant surgery may be an option for someone with significant hearing impairment, but is not considered to fix the problem as it does not repair the damaged cochlea; rather, it uses a different method to stimulate the vestibulocochlear nerve. The range of hearing loss with a sensorineural problem can be from slight to profound. Clients with sensorineural hearing loss often have more trouble hearing clearly as the hair cells in the cochlea are often damaged. A client with a sensorineural hearing loss may be able to hear that you are talking, but may not be able to understand the words or the sounds of words easily. If you asked a client to tell you about a cat and they started describing that you would use it to hit a ball, as a clinician you would count this as incorrect; whereas, the client may have heard you ask to describe what you would do with a bat.

Hearing loss can affect speech/language skills in a variety of ways. If you do not have an accurate picture of your client's hearing, you cannot rule out hearing loss as a possible cause for their communication difficulties.

When

Hearing should be screened prior to a speech/language evaluation. If the client has had a recent hearing screen (typically one year or less), it may be acceptable to use those results. Keep in mind, however, hearing loss, particularly conductive loss, can come on rapidly. It is also very possible for someone to have a permanent hearing loss that they do not recognize; therefore, he/she would not be inclined to report it because a permanent hearing loss can be gradual and a person would not even realize they do not hear as well.

Best case scenario would be to screen hearing the day of the evaluation. Hearing screenings do not typically take a long time to complete. Making sure the client is hearing at a level that allows them to understand the questions you are asking will ensure you have valid and reliable results.

Where

Ideally, hearing screenings will be completed in a quiet environment. Depending on the location of your testing, this may not always happen. If you are testing at a busy school, hospital, skilled nursing facility, or other location where you may not have a room to yourself to test, you may have to deal with some additional background noise. In these cases, you may have to adjust your screening levels. If this occurs, you want to make sure you are screening at a level where you do not have an increased chance of false positives (saying someone has a hearing loss when they do not) or false negatives (passing individuals who actually have a hearing loss). Typically, the clinician would screen at intensity (or loudness) levels of 20 to 25 dB (decibels); however, if there are high levels of background noise and the client would fail the screening, not because they have a hearing loss but because the background noise would interfere, you may need to raise the screening level. It is important that clinicians are familiar with their own hearing levels so you can do a listening check before you screen. By knowing if you can normally hear a 20 dB tone with no problems yet you are struggling when you are performing your listening check prior to screening, you would likely need to raise your screening level to hear over the background noise.

How

Audiological equipment, including audiometers, used for testing must be calibrated annually (Occupational Safety and Health Administration, n.d.). If you are not sure if the equipment has been calibrated, you should not use that piece of equipment. Calibrations ensure that your equipment is indeed presenting tones at frequencies/intensities that correspond to the frequency/intensity you are selecting. Daily visual and listening checks should also be done. Prior to using the equipment for the day, you must make sure there are no loose knobs or cords and you should run through the frequencies and intensities to make sure things seem to be in proper working condition (Health and Safety Authority, n.d.).

While most states do not have hearing screening requirements, there are recommendations. The idea behind a hearing screening is that you will be able to detect if there is a problem outside the range of normal hearing. This means you do not have to know how soft they can hear, only that they are hearing within normal limits. You will want to cover a range of frequencies (or pitches). Many recommendations include screening 1000 hertz (Hz), 2000 Hz, 4000 Hz, and perhaps one of the higher frequencies such as 6000 Hz or 8000 Hz. However, many recommendations do not include screening at 500 Hz as it is often compromised in background noise. Remember that the majority of the speech frequencies are between 1000 to 4000 Hz; thus, if a person is hearing normally for those frequencies, they should not have any problems hearing your instructions or conversation during the speech/language evaluation.

In some circumstances, a person will not tolerate the headphones for testing or may not be able to respond consistently to the stimuli even though they hear it. In these cases, it is important to know how you will determine if proceeding with the speech/language evaluation without a hearing screening is acceptable. Oftentimes, clinicians will use the interview part of the evaluation to determine gross hearing ability. This means that the clinician will be able to report that during normal conversation the client was able to hear, understand, and respond appropriately to normal conversation levels. Using this method does not validate hearing to be within normal limits but may indicate that the client had no difficulty hearing normal conversational speech levels so testing in a quiet environment at normal conversational levels should be appropriate.

When you complete hearing screenings, you should get as much information as possible. This means you should ideally screen at the predetermined frequencies (for instance, the frequencies listed previously), at the predetermined level (20 dB or 25 dB, unless adjustments need to be made due to background noise), and for each ear. A hearing screening is different than determining hearing thresholds (the softest level a client can consistently hear), because you present a tone and the client either hears the tone or does not. For most screenings, a fail at any frequency for either ear constitutes a fail and the client should be referred for further testing. As a clinician, you will have to determine if you will move forward with testing if the client fails the hearing screening. There may be instances where the client fails the screening but hears adequately in a quiet environment at normal conversational levels so you may continue with the speech/language evaluation and recommend that the client follow up for further hearing testing.

When screening, it is important to keep in mind the age, cognitive abilities, attention span, and speech/language abilities of the client. If the client is very young, it is highly unlikely they will be able to listen to tones and respond by pressing a button or raising his/her hand. The clinician may need to make the screening more of a gamelike activity, such as throwing blocks in a bucket when they hear the tone. If a client has cognitive impairments, such as dementia, the clinician may need to adapt testing by giving written directions or slowing down their rate of speech when giving instructions, repeating instructions often, or determining appropriate response methods (e.g., raising a finger, watching for changes in eye movement or facial expressions, having the client say "yes" when they hear the tone) (Polovoy, 2017). It is most important to obtain reliable and valid results when screening hearing, regardless of the method that is used to reach those results.

Top 10 Terms

Frequency

Intensity

Decibel/dB

Hertz/Hz

Threshold

Screening

False positive

False negative

Calibration

Listening check

Chapter Tips

1. Hearing problems can lead to speech and/or language problems. Prior to determining if a speech/language problem is present, you want to identify if there is a hearing loss that could be contributing to the problem.

2. Best practice is to screen hearing prior to the speech/language evaluation. While it may be acceptable to use hearing screening or evaluation results obtained within one year of your testing, it is highly possible that you could miss a hearing component that could be causing a speech/language problem or could impede results in treatment.

3. Any equipment used to screen hearing must be calibrated annually and a listening/visual check should be done daily when you are using the equipment. Calibration and daily checks ensures that your equipment is working the way you think it is and that you are not getting false information when screening.

Activities

12–1. Use the following scenarios to complete the hearing screening form (provided in Figure 12–1) and write up your results for the hearing section of your evaluation.

Scenario #1

Mary Mack is your client. Mary's date of birth is 03-01-1929. The date of your screening is 01-15-2020. Mary passed the screening using 25 dB at 1000 Hz and 2000 Hz for the right and left ears; she did not pass 4000 Hz or 8000 Hz for either ear. She did not struggle to hear you during the interview portion of the test.

Write-up for report:

_____

_____

_____

_____

Hearing Screening Form

Name: _____ Date of Birth: _____
Date of Screening: _____

	1000 Hz	2000 Hz	4000 Hz	6000 Hz	8000 Hz
Right ear					
Left ear					

P = Pass

R = Refer

DNT = Did not test

Intensity level = 20 dB unless otherwise noted here
_____

Recommendation:
_____
_____

Clinician Name:
_____

Figure 12–1. Hearing screening form. This is a sample hearing screening form that could be used for all ages screened.

Scenario #2

Johnny Jumper is your client. Johnny's date of birth is 07-01-2010. The date of your screening is 10-01-2017. Johnny passed the screening using 20 dB at 1000 Hz, 2000 Hz, 4000 Hz, and 6000 Hz for the right ear, and 2000 Hz, 4000 Hz, and 6000 Hz for the left ear. During the interview Johnny reported his left ear had been hurting.

Write-up for report:

_____
_____
_____
_____

12–2. Determine if the following statements are true or false.

____ 1. A "refer" (or fail) for any frequency at either ear indicates a failed hearing screening.

___ 2. It is not necessary to determine hearing to be adequate for normal conversational speech prior to speech/language testing.

___ 3. Listening/visual checks on the audiometer should be done daily when being used for screenings.

___ 4. A person must have passed a hearing screening prior to testing for speech/language problems.

___ 5. You must test all possible frequencies when completing a hearing screening.

Answers to Activities

12–1.

Hearing Screening Form

Name: Mary Mack   Date of Birth: 3-1-29

Date of Screening: 01-15-20

	1000 Hz	2000 Hz	4000 Hz	6000 Hz	8000 Hz
Right ear	P	P	R	DNT	R
Left ear	P	P	R	DNT	R

P = Pass

R = Refer

DNT = Did not test

Intensity level = 20 dB unless otherwise noted here
25 dB

Recommendation:
Did not pass screening for high frequencies at either ear. A complete hearing evaluation is recommended.

Clinician Name:
Tracie Rice

Figure 12–2. Sample completed hearing screening form using information from Activity 12–1, scenario #1.

Write-up for report: Hearing screening results indicate Ms. Mack did not pass the higher frequencies on the hearing screening. Ms. Mack did not have difficulty hearing normal conversational levels during the interview section of the evaluation. Ms. Mack's hearing was considered to be adequate for testing purposes at normal conversational levels in a quiet environment; thus, testing was completed. It is recommended she follow up for a complete hearing evaluation.

Hearing Screening Form

Name: Johnny Jumper   Date of Birth: 7-1-10

Date of Screening: 10-1-17

	1000 Hz	2000 Hz	4000 Hz	6000 Hz	8000 Hz
Right ear	P	P	P	P	DNT
Left ear	R	P	P	P	DNT

P = Pass

R = Refer

DNT = Did not test

Intensity level = 20 dB unless otherwise noted here
_____

Recommendation:
Did not pass screening for left ear. Complained of ear ache in his left ear. Follow-up with doctor.

Clinician Name:
Tracie Rice

Figure 12–3. Sample completed hearing screening form using information from Activity 12–1, scenario #2.

Write-up for report: Hearing screening results indicate Johnny did not pass the hearing screening for the left ear. During the interview portion, Johnny indicated his left ear was hurting. He did not appear to have difficulty hearing normal conversation levels and hearing was judged to be adequate for speech/language testing at normal conversational levels in a quiet environment. It is recommended Johnny follow up with his doctor due to the failed hearing screening and pain in his left ear.

12–2.

1. **True.** A refer for any frequency at either ear indicates a failed hearing screening.
2. **False.** It is not necessary to determine hearing to be adequate for normal conversational speech prior to speech/language testing. (You should always determine that hearing is adequate for normal conversational levels prior to testing for speech/language problems.)
3. **True.** Listening/visual checks on the audiometer should be done daily when being used for screenings.
4. **False.** A person must have passed a hearing screening prior to testing for speech/language problems. (While a person does not necessarily have to pass a hearing screening, you as the clinician should judge that the person's hearing is adequate for hearing normal conversational speech in a quiet environment prior to testing.)

5. **False.** You must test all possible frequencies when completing a hearing screening. (You should screen a variety of frequencies, but do not have to screen every frequency.)

Wrap-Up

Things do not always go as planned when we are screening hearing or testing for speech/language problems. Think about if you were not be able to continue with speech/language testing based on hearing screening results. What would be your recommendations? How would your write-up/screening process change if someone comes to the evaluation wearing hearing aids? Would a person who already wears hearing aids be able to pass a hearing screening? What steps would you take to verify the person is able to hear at normal conversation levels in a quiet environment?

_____

_____

_____

_____

References

Health and Safety Authority. (n.d.). Guidelines on hearing checks and audiometry under the safety, health and welfare at work. Retrieved October 29, 2017, from http://www.hsa.ie/eng/Publications_and_Forms/Publications/Occupational_Health/audio metry.pdf

Lin, F. R., Metter, E. J., O'Brien, R. J., Resnick, S. M., Zonderman, A. B., & Ferrucci, L. (2011). Hearing loss and incident dementia. *Archives of Neurology, 68*(2):214–220.

Madell, J. R., & Flexer, C. (2014). *Pediatric audiology: Diagnosis, technology, and management* (2nd ed.). New York, NY: Thieme.

Occupational Safety and Health Administration. (n.d.). Regulations. Retrieved October 19, 2017, from https://www.osha.gov/pls/oshaweb/owadisp.show_document?p_table=STANDARDS&p_id=9740

Polovoy, C. (2017). Cognitive impairment and hearing assessment. *The ASHA Leader, 22*(8), 62.

CHAPTER 13

Billing

Who

Clinicians need at least a basic understanding of billing issues and practices. In order to be paid for services, clinicians must understand how to code a visit or procedure as well as assign the appropriate diagnostic code for the client. Oftentimes, there is someone within the practice or entity you work for who has an education and a background in billing; however, in some instances, you may be responsible for turning in your billing and procedure codes to the owner or even a billing company or payment source if you are the owner. Clinicians must remember that whatever contains their signature or license number is ultimately their responsibility. Because of this, clinicians want to make sure they are using the highest ethical standards, which includes at least a basic understanding of billing issues. It is important to note that billing codes are not written in stone and do change, sometimes as often as annually. Some great examples of this are the changes for the year 2018 that include a new cognitive therapy code that should replace an old code as well as the changes to Medicare in which the therapy caps are lifted (Swanson, 2018). There are great online resources that provide updated billing/coding information as it is discussed and approved by the insurance and billing regulators (American Speech-Language-Hearing Association, n.d.).

What

A good starting point is understanding the differences between the three main billing coding systems we use. The International Classification of Diseases, 10th Revision, Clinical Modification (ICD-10 CM) is the system we use for diagnostic codes. The intent is to standardize the classification of diseases and disorders. This system uses alpha-numeric identification and is much more specific than previously used systems. The first character is a letter with numbers and/or letters following (International Classification of Diseases-10th Revision-Clinical Modification, n.d.). The code could be as short as three characters or as long as seven characters. Typically, the longer the code, the more specific the description is. For example, F84 is for pervasive developmental disorders, but to be more specific, autism is F84.0 and Asperger's syndrome is F84.5 (International Classification of Diseases-10th Revision- Clinical Modification, n.d.). When coding, clinicians should keep in mind that a client can have more than one diagnosis code. Clinicians should use the speech-language code as the primary code and then other medical diagnoses as additional codes. An example of this might be a client with multiple sclerosis receiving treatment for dysphagia. The primary code would be R13.10 for dysphagia unspecified with G35 for multiple sclerosis as a secondary code. One question that clinicians often have is, "What code do I use if the client tests as normal?" In this case, you would use the code that describes what you are evaluating. So, if the doctor referral asked for you to evaluate due to language delays, you could use F80.2, which is mixed expressive/receptive language disorder.

The next set of codes used are the Current Procedural Terminology (CPT) codes. These codes are used to describe what services are completed. These codes are published and maintained by the American Medical Association (n.d) (AMA) and are five numeric characters in length (e.g., 92507: treatment of speech, language, swallowing, voice, communication, or auditory processing disorder/individual). For speech-language pathologists, there are not as many CPT codes as ICD-10 codes that we often deal with. For instance, the above listed code, 92507, is the most common code for individual speech-language treatment. There are a variety of evaluation codes depending on the type of evaluation you are conducting, such as speech sound production only (92522) or evaluation of speech sound production with language comprehension and expression (92523). The American Speech-Language-Hearing Association (ASHA) has many helpful and simple-to-understand resources such as a model superbill that lists the possible CPT codes one may use in this profession. In rare instances, clinicians may also find the need to use a modifier while coding. Most modifiers are two digit numbers added to the end of the CPT code using a hyphen. These are often used to provide additional information to the code. When the procedure takes substantially longer to complete, the -22 modifier is used; whereas, if the procedure is not fully completed, the -52 modifier is used.

The final set of codes that should be discussed are the Healthcare Common Procedures Coding System (HCPCS; often called "hick picks"). These codes are five-character, alpha-numeric codes that are used to describe procedures not otherwise covered through the CPT codes. Primarily in speech pathology and audiology we use these codes for durable medical equipment, supplies, devices, and services not found in the CPT codes. Equipment such as Augmentative and Alternative Communication (AAC) devices and hearing aids are coded using HCPCS codes.

Why

Billing must be done ethically and accurately. While speech-language pathologists and audiologists will likely not be primarily responsible for knowing billing procedures in most work environments, we do have a professional and ethical obligation to be familiar with coding practices and ensure correct information is provided. Ultimately, as a clinician, your license will be on the line. In order to make sure your client's welfare is held paramount, you must know that you are providing the services you are billing for.

Although we have set codes and guidelines to use, it is important to keep in mind that various agencies and pay sources may have certain requirements that must be followed when coding. Not all services that have a code will be covered. As clinicians, you may find yourself working with agencies and payment sources to determine their specific requirements in order to get reimbursement for services. Not all agencies pay for all procedure codes or even diagnosis codes. Learning the specific guidelines takes time; however, starting with a general understanding of coding policies and practices will help you learn the additional specifics. It is not uncommon for speech pathologists to encounter situations with insurance companies that will only pay for certain services or types of treatment (i.e., some insurances will deny speech treatment for autism and claim that they will only pay for applied behavior analysis [ABA]). When situations like this arise, it is important for the speech pathologist to be aware of laws that prohibit insurance companies from dictating the type of treatment that is given, as individuals respond to certain services and it is up to the trained professional to determine what is best (Havens, 2017). It may be up to the speech-language pathologist to contact the insurance company and refer to policies that are in place to make sure patients are receiving the most beneficial services for them and their disorder.

While this chapter covers the three main coding systems used in this field, please know this is not all-inclusive. For instance, specific codes such as G-Codes, which are modifiers that are used with Medicare Part B to determine severity/complexity of problems, are not discussed. Once again, ASHA has very easy to understand information for providers and clinicians should take the time to review this information for a better understanding.

When

Billing is completed after the session concludes. Clinicians may have information before the session, such as what the referral source is asking for (e.g., an evaluation of speech sound disorders, swallowing difficulties, voice concerns, etc.); however, the clinician must determine what is best practice as well as what information may be required from some agencies. An example could be that you have been given a referral for a child with speech sound production errors and asked to evaluate and treat. The child is school aged, but the parents are requesting an evaluation to be completed by an outside (other than school) source. Although the referral speaks directly about speech sound production, as a clinician, you know the school system will also need some information on the child's language abilities. As a clinician, you may choose to evaluate both the speech and language skills of the child. You would then choose a billing code that represents the actual procedures you performed. You will also want to make sure you are using the correct ICD-10 codes after seeing the client and determining what codes are appropriate for that individual. Remember, you will use the code that best represents the cause or diagnosis of the speech/language concern, but you may have multiple codes and additional medical codes to add to the primary speech/language code. If you are working with some type of medical durable equipment or services, you may also be using HCPCS codes.

Where

Coding information may be found or used with a variety of forms. Many offices have a billing form that has commonly used codes listed. Figure 13–1 is an example of a superbill that has codes that are most often used within a particular practice. This superbill does not have all the codes; however, additional codes could always be added.

Speech and Hearing Clinic (CHARGE CAPTURE)

Patient Full Name _____ Patient DOB _____
Patient Address _____
City, State, Zip _____
Patient Phone _____ PROVIDER _____
Referring Physician _____
Insurance Carrier _____ Patient PMT$ _____
Insurance ID _____
Preauthorization# _____

HEARING DIAGNOSIS

H90.6 Mixed;bilateral	H90.0 Conductive hearing loss; bilateral	H93.25 Auditory Processing Dis
H90.71 mixed;unilat right	H90.11 Conductive hearing loss; right	H91.23 Sudden hearing loss
H90.72 mixed; unilat left	H90.12 Conductive hearing loss; left	H83.3x9 Noise induced hrng loss
Z01.10 hearing screen	H90.3 Sensorineural hearing loss	F45.8 Functional hearing loss

HEARING CHARGES

Testing

92551	Pass/Fail "Screening"
92555	Speech audiometry threshold
92556	Speech audiometry threshold w/ recog
92557	Comprehensive Audiometry Threshold
92567	Tympanometry;middle ear/eardrum test
92582	Conditioned Play Audiometry
92587	Distortion emission;3-11 frequencies per ear

DEVICES/PROGRAMMING

V5011	HA fitting/orientation
V5014	Repair/Modification/Adjust
V5110	Dispensing Fee
V5253	HA;Digital; Binaural BTE
V5264	Ear mold; non-disposable
V5275	Ear impression; each

Evaluations

92626	Hearing Aid Testing(Rehab status); 60 min
92620	Eval w/ Report;Central Auditory; 60 min
92625	Tinnitus Assessment(pitch/loud/masking)

SPEECH DIAGNOSIS

F80.1 Expressive Lng. Dis	I69.990 Apraxia Following Unspec CVA	R47.0 Aphasia	F84.0 Autism
F80.2 Mixed Exp/Rec Lgn Dis	R13.14 Dysphagia	R47.1 Dysarthria	F98.5 Fluency; adulthd onset
F80.0 Phonology Dis.	I69.992 Facial Weakness following CVA	R49.2 Dysphonia	F80.81 Fluency; childhd onset

SPEECH CHARGES

Testing/Evaluation Charges

92521	Speech Fluency Eval(eg. Stuttering)
92522	Speech Sound Production(eg. Articualtion)
92523	Speech Sound Production w/ Language comprehension and expressive evaluation
92524	Behavioral and qualitative analysis of voice and resonance

Treatment Charges

92507	Tx of speech, lang., voice, communication and/or auditory disorder; individual
92508	Tx of speech, lang., voice, communication and/or auditory disorder; group

CATEGORY	CURRENT	GOAL	DISCHARGE	IMPAIRMENT LVL	
Speech	G8999____	G9186____	G9158____	CI	1-19%
Compreh.	G9159____	G9160____	G9161____	CJ	20-39%
Expression	G9162____	G9163____	G9164____	CK	40-59%
Voice	G9171____	G9172____	G9173____	CL	60-79%

Figure 13–1. Superbill that has codes that are most often used within a particular practice.

Billing information must also be sent to insurance companies. Sometimes billing information is sent electronically or by using a 3rd party billing company or clearinghouse. In these instances, information may be inputted electronically into a particular form or portal. There are also paper billing forms that may be required. One example of this is called a HCFA 1500 pronounced "Hicfa 1500." This form is often required for Medicare/Medicaid billing; other state agencies and private insurances use this form as well. An example of a blank HCFA 1500 is provided in Figure 13–2.

Figure 13–2. Example of a blank HCFA 1500 form. (*continues*)

BECAUSE THIS FORM IS USED BY VARIOUS GOVERNMENT AND PRIVATE HEALTH PROGRAMS, SEE SEPARATE INSTRUCTIONS ISSUED BY APPLICABLE PROGRAMS.

NOTICE: Any person who knowingly files a statement of claim containing any misrepresentation or any false, incomplete or misleading information may be guilty of a criminal act punishable under law and may be subject to civil penalties.

REFERS TO GOVERNMENT PROGRAMS ONLY

MEDICARE AND TRICARE PAYMENTS: A patient's signature requests that payment be made and authorizes release of any information necessary to process the claim and certifies that the information provided in Blocks 1 through 12 is true, accurate and complete. In the case of a Medicare claim, the patient's signature authorizes any entity to release to Medicare medical and nonmedical information and whether the person has employer group health insurance, liability, no-fault, worker's compensation or other insurance which is responsible to pay for the services for which the Medicare claim is made. See 42 CFR 411.24(a). If item 9 is completed, the patient's signature authorizes release of the information to the health plan or agency shown. In Medicare assigned or TRICARE participation cases, the physician agrees to accept the charge determination of the Medicare carrier or TRICARE fiscal intermediary as the full charge and the patient is responsible only for the deductible, coinsurance and non-covered services. Coinsurance and the deductible are based upon the charge determination of the Medicare carrier or TRICARE fiscal intermediary if this is less than the charge submitted. TRICARE is not a health insurance program but makes payment for health benefits provided through certain affiliations with the Uniformed Services. Information on the patient's sponsor should be provided in those items captioned in "Insured"; i.e., items 1a, 4, 6, 7, 9 and 11.

BLACK LUNG AND FECA CLAIMS

The provider agrees to accept the amount paid by the Government as payment in full. See Black Lung and FECA instructions regarding required procedure and diagnosis coding systems.

SIGNATURE OF PHYSICIAN OR SUPPLIER (MEDICARE, TRICARE, FECA AND BLACK LUNG)

In submitting this claim for payment from federal funds, I certify that: 1) the information on this form is true, accurate and complete, 2) I have familiarized myself with all applicable laws, regulations, and program instructions, which are available from the Medicare contractor; 3) I have provided or will provide sufficient information required to allow the government to make an informed eligibility and payment decision; 4) this claim, whether submitted by me or on my behalf by my designated billing company, complies with all applicable Medicare and/or Medicaid laws, regulations, and program instructions for payment including but not limited to the Federal anti-kickback statute and Physician Self-Referral law (commonly known as Stark law), 5) the services on this form were medically necessary and personally furnished by me or were furnished incident to my professional service by my employee under my direct supervision, except as otherwise expressly permitted by Medicare or TRICARE; 6) for each service rendered incident to my professional service, the identity (legal name and NPI, license #, or SSN) of the primary individual rendering each service is reported in the designated section. For services to be considered "incident to" a physician's professional services, 1) they must be rendered under the physician's direct supervision by his/her employee, 2) they must be an integral, although incidental part of a covered physician service, 3) they must be of kinds commonly furnished in physician's offices, and 4) the services of non-physicians must be included on the physician's bills.

For TRICARE claims, I further certify that I (or any employee) who rendered services am not an active duty member of the Uniformed Services or a civilian employee of the United States Government or a contract employee of the United States Government, either civilian or military (refer to 5 USC 5536). For Black-Lung claims, I further certify that the services performed were for a Black Lung-related disorder.

No Part B Medicare benefits may be paid unless this form is received as required by existing law and regulations (42 CFR 424.32).

NOTICE: Any one who misrepresents or falsifies essential information to receive payment from Federal funds requested by this form may upon conviction be subject to fine and imprisonment under applicable Federal laws.

NOTICE TO PATIENT ABOUT THE COLLECTION AND USE OF MEDICARE, TRICARE, FECA, AND BLACK LUNG INFORMATION (PRIVACY ACT STATEMENT)

We are authorized by CMS, TRICARE and OWCP to ask you for information needed in the administration of the Medicare, TRICARE, FECA, and Black Lung programs. Authority to collect information is in section 205(a), 1862, 1872 and 1874 of the Social Security Act as amended, 42 CFR 411.24(a) and 424.5(a) (6), and 44 USC 3101,41 CFR 101 et seq and 10 USC 1079 and 1086; 5 USC 8101 et seq; and 30 USC 901 et seq; 38 USC 613; E.O. 9397.

The information we obtain to complete claims under these programs is used to identify you and to determine your eligibility. It is also used to decide if the services and supplies you received are covered by these programs and to insure that proper payment is made.

The information may also be given to other providers of services, carriers, intermediaries, medical review boards, health plans, and other organizations or Federal agencies, for the effective administration of Federal provisions that require other third parties payers to pay primary to Federal program, and as otherwise necessary to administer these programs. For example, it may be necessary to disclose information about the benefits you have used to a hospital or doctor. Additional disclosures are made through routine uses for information contained in systems of records.

FOR MEDICARE CLAIMS: See the notice modifying system No. 09-70-0501, titled, 'Carrier Medicare Claims Record,' published in the Federal Register, Vol 55 No. 177, page 37549, Wed. Sept. 12, 1990, or as updated and republished.

FOR OWCP CLAIMS: Department of Labor, Privacy Act of 1974, "Republication of Notice of Systems of Records," Federal Register Vol. 55 No. 40, Wed Feb 28, 1990, See ESA-5, ESA-6, ESA-12, ESA-13, ESA-30, or as updated and republished.

FOR TRICARE CLAIMS: PRINCIPLE PURPOSE(S): To evaluate eligibility for medical care provided by civilian sources and to issue payment upon establishment of eligibility and determination that the services/supplies received are authorized by law

ROUTINE USE(S): Information from claims and related documents may be given to the Dept. of Veterans Affairs, the Dept. of Health and Human Services and/or the Dept of Transportation consistent with their statutory administrative responsibilities under TRICARE/CHAMPVA, to the Dept. of Justice for representation of the Secretary of Defense in civil actions; to the Internal Revenue Service, private collection agencies, and consumer reporting agencies in connection with recoupment claims; and to Congressional Offices in response to inquiries made at the request of the person to whom a record pertains. Appropriate disclosures may be made to other federal, state, local, foreign government agencies, private business entities, and individual providers of care, on matters relating to entitlement, claims adjudication, fraud, program abuse, utilization review, quality assurance, peer review, program integrity, third-party liability, coordination of benefits, and civil and criminal litigation related to the operation of TRICARE.

DISCLOSURES: Voluntary; however, failure to provide information will result in delay in payment or may result in denial of claim. With the one exception discussed below, there are no penalties under these programs for refusing to supply information. However, failure to furnish information regarding the medical services rendered or the amount charged would prevent payment of claims under these programs. Failure to furnish any other information, such as name or claim number, would delay payment of the claim. Failure to provide medical information under FECA could be deemed an obstruction.

It is mandatory that you tell us if you know that another party is responsible for paying for your treatment. Section 1128B of the Social Security Act and 31 USC 3801-3812 provide penalties for withholding this information.

You should be aware that P.L. 100-503, the "Computer Matching and Privacy Protection Act of 1988", permits the government to verify information by way of computer matches.

MEDICAID PAYMENTS (PROVIDER CERTIFICATION)

I hereby agree to keep such records as are necessary to disclose fully the extent of services provided to individuals under the State's Title XIX plan and to furnish information regarding any payments claimed for providing such services as the State Agency or Dept of Health and Human Services may request.

I further agree to accept, as payment in full, the amount paid by the Medicaid program for those claims submitted for payment under that program with the exception of authorized deductible, coinsurance, co-payment or similar cost-sharing charge.

SIGNATURE OF PHYSICIAN (OR SUPPLIER): I certify that the services listed above were medically indicated and necessary to the health of this patient and were personally furnished by me or my employee under my personal direction.

NOTICE: This is to certify that the foregoing information is true, accurate and complete. I understand that payment and satisfaction of this claim will be from Federal and State funds, and that any false claims, statements, or documents, or concealment of a material fact, may be prosecuted under applicable Federal or State laws.

According to the Paperwork Reduction Act of 1995, no persons are required to respond to a collection of information unless it displays a valid OMB control number. The valid OMB control number for this information collection is 0938-1197. The time required to complete this information collection is estimated to average 10 minutes per response, including the time to review instructions, search existing data resources, gather the data needed, and complete and review the information collection. If you have any comments concerning the accuracy of the time estimate(s) or suggestions for improving this form, please write to: CMS, 7500 Security Boulevard, Attn: PRA Reports Clearance Officer, Mail Stop C4-26-05 Baltimore, Maryland 21244-1850. This address is for comments and/or suggestions only. DO NOT MAIL COMPLETED CLAIM FORMS TO THIS ADDRESS.

Figure 13–2. (*continued*)

How

Billing should always be completed as thoroughly and accurately as possible. Having a person who is trained in billing procedures is a wonderful resource, but may not always be available in every practice. Using the highest level of coding is required by payer sources as well as state licensing authorities. There are several resources available to clinicians to assist in understanding and proper use of coding strategies.

Top 10 Terms

Coding

ICD-10

CPT codes

HCPCS codes

HCFA 1500

G-Codes

Diagnosis codes

Procedure codes

Durable medical equipment

Duperbill

Chapter Tips

1. It is your responsibility as a clinician to be knowledgeable regarding proper coding procedures.
2. There are many resources available to help guide you through the coding and billing process.
3. Coding strategies vary from agency to agency and may change over time. For instance, the ICD-10 codes are only a few years old and are revisited annually so there are often changes that occur that you as the clinician are responsible for knowing.

Activities

13–1. Using the model superbill in Figure 13–3, determine the correct ICD-10 and CPT codes for a fluency evaluation with a person who has recently started stuttering following their 40th birthday.

Speech and Hearing Clinic (CHARGE CAPTURE)

Patient Full Name: _____ Patient DOB: _____
Patient Address: _____
City, State, Zip: _____
Patient Phone: _____ PROVIDER: _____
Referring Physician: _____
Insurance Carrier: _____ Patient PMT$: _____
Insurance ID: _____
Preauthorization#: _____

HEARING DIAGNOSIS

H90.6 Mixed;bilateral	H90.0 Conductive hearing loss; bilateral	H93.25 Auditory Processing Dis
H90.71 mixed;unilat right	H90.11 Conductive hearing loss; right	H91.23 Sudden hearing loss
H90.72 mixed; unilat left	H90.12 Conductive hearing loss; left	H83.3x9 Noise induced hrng loss
Z01.10 hearing screen	H90.3 Sensorineural hearing loss	F45.8 Functional hearing loss

HEARING CHARGES

Testing | DEVICES/PROGRAMMING

Code	Testing	Code	Devices/Programming
92551	Pass/Fail "Screening"	V5011	HA fitting/orientation
92555	Speech audiometry threshold	V5014	Repair/Modification/Adjust
92556	Speech audiometry threshold w/ recog	V5110	Dispensing Fee
92557	Comprehensive Audiometry Threshold	V5253	HA;Digital; Binaural BTE
92567	Tympanometry;middle ear/eardrum test	V5264	Ear mold; non-disposable
92582	Conditioned Play Audiometry	V5275	Ear impression; each
92587	Distortion emission;3-11 frequencies per ear		

Evaluations

92626	Hearing Aid Testing(Rehab status); 60 min
92620	Eval w/ Report;Central Auditory; 60 min
92625	Tinnitus Assessment(pitch/loud/masking)

SPEECH DIAGNOSIS

F80.1 Expressive Lng. Dis	I69.990 Apraxia Following Unspec CVA	R47.0 Aphasia	F84.0 Autism
F80.2 Mixed Exp/Rec Lgn Dis	R13.14 Dysphagia	R47.1 Dysarthria	F98.5 Fluency; adulthd onset
F80.0 Phonology Dis.	I69.992 Facial Weakness following CVA	R49.2 Dysphonia	F80.81 Fluency; childhd onset

SPEECH CHARGES

Testing/Evaluation Charges

92521	Speech Fluency Eval(eg. Stuttering)
92522	Speech Sound Production(eg. Articualtion)
92523	Speech Sound Production w/ Language comprehension and expressive evaluation
92524	Behavioral and qualitative analysis of voice and resonance

Treatment Charges

92507	Tx of speech, lang., voice, communication and/or auditory disorder; individual
92508	Tx of speech, lang., voice, communication and/or auditory disorder; group

CATEGORY	CURRENT	GOAL	DISCHARGE	IMPAIRMENT LVL	
Speech	G8999____	G9186____	G9158____	CI	1-19%
Compreh.	G9159____	G9160____	G9161____	CJ	20-39%
Expression	G9162____	G9163____	G9164____	CK	40-59%
Voice	G9171____	G9172____	G9173____	CL	60-79%

Figure 13–3. Model superbill for Activity 13–1.

13–2. Using the model superbill in Figure 13–4, determine the correct ICD-10 and CPT codes for a speech/language evaluation with a child who has no other medical issues but has been referred due to not being able to be understood by familiar listeners and difficulty following directions.

Speech and Hearing Clinic (CHARGE CAPTURE)

Patient Full Name	Patient DOB _____
Patient Address	
City, State, Zip	
Patient Phone	PROVIDER _____
Referring Physician	
Insurance Carrier	Patient PMT$ _____
Insurance ID	
Preauthorization#	

HEARING DIAGNOSIS

H90.6 Mixed;bilateral	H90.0 Conductive hearing loss; bilateral	H93.25 Auditory Processing Dis
H90.71 mixed;unilat right	H90.11 Conductive hearing loss; right	H91.23 Sudden hearing loss
H90.72 mixed; unilat left	H90.12 Conductive hearing loss; left	H83.3x9 Noise induced hrng loss
Z01.10 hearing screen	H90.3 Sensorineural hearing loss	F45.8 Functional hearing loss

HEARING CHARGES

Testing | DEVICES/PROGRAMMING

92551	Pass/Fail "Screening"	V5011	HA fitting/orientation
92555	Speech audiometry threshold	V5014	Repair/Modification/Adjust
92556	Speech audiometry threshold w/ recog	V5110	Dispensing Fee
92557	Comprehensive Audiometry Threshold	V5253	HA;Digital; Binaural BTE
92567	Tympanometry;middle ear/eardrum test	V5264	Ear mold; non-disposable
92582	Conditioned Play Audiometry	V5275	Ear impression; each
92587	Distortion emission;3-11 frequencies per ear		

Evaluations

92626	Hearing Aid Testing(Rehab status); 60 min
92620	Eval w/ Report;Central Auditory; 60 min
92625	Tinnitus Assessment(pitch/loud/masking)

SPEECH DIAGNOSIS

F80.1 Expressive Lng. Dis	I69.990 Apraxia Following Unspec CVA	R47.0 Aphasia	F84.0 Autism
F80.2 Mixed Exp/Rec Lgn Dis	R13.14 Dysphagia	R47.1 Dysarthria	F98.5 Fluency; adulthd onset
F80.0 Phonology Dis.	I69.992 Facial Weakness following CVA	R49.2 Dysphonia	F80.81 Fluency; childhd onset

SPEECH CHARGES

Testing/Evaluation Charges

92521	Speech Fluency Eval(eg. Stuttering)
92522	Speech Sound Production(eg. Articualtion)
92523	Speech Sound Production w/ Language comprehension and expressive evaluation
92524	Behavioral and qualitative analysis of voice and resonance

Treatment Charges

92507	Tx of speech, lang., voice, communication and/or auditory disorder; individual
92508	Tx of speech, lang., voice, communication and/or auditory disorder; group

CATEGORY	CURRENT	GOAL	DISCHARGE	IMPAIRMENT LVL	
Speech	G8999____	G9186____	G9158____	CI	1-19%
Compreh.	G9159____	G9160____	G9161____	CJ	20-39%
Expression	G9162____	G9163____	G9164____	CK	40-59%
Voice	G9171____	G9172____	G9173____	CL	60-79%

Figure 13–4. Model superbill for Activity 13–2.

13–3. Match the following terms:

____**1.** A set of codes used to describe services that are not otherwise covered by the Current Procedural Terminology codes. These may be related to durable medical equipment, services, or other equipment used with a client.

___ **2.** A series of five numeric characters to determine the activities or services that were provided.

___ **3.** A combination of alpha-numeric numbers ranging from three to seven characters to describe the cause or reason a client is receiving services.

A. ICD-10 codes

B. CPT codes

C. HCPCS codes

Answers to Activities

13–1. ICD-10 code: F98.5
CPT code: 92521

13–2. ICD-10 code: F80.2
CPT code: 92523

13–3. 1 = C, 2 = B, 3 = A

Wrap-Up

1. Think about your life after graduate school as a speech-language pathologist. Imagine you are going to an interview. One question that will always be asked is, "Do you have any questions for us?" Think about three possible questions you could ask regarding billing practices within the company (your responsibilities, company policies and procedures, training modules, etc.). List them in the following spaces.

   Question 1:
   _____
   _____
   _____
   _____

   Question 2:
   _____
   _____
   _____
   _____

Question 3:

2. Review websites such as those listed in the reference section. What concepts do you feel you understand well? What concepts do you require additional information? Find a YouTube video on practices for billing for the speech pathologist. Did this bring up new questions?

3. Search for information for the state in which you plan to be licensed. Are there certain billing issues specific to the state? What are specific billing issues related to the school systems versus private practice or medical setting?

References

American Medical Assocation (n.d.). Medical coding vocabulary & key terms. Retrieved November 28, 2017, from http://www.medicalbillingandcoding.org/coding-vocabulary-key-terms/

American Speech-Language-Hearing Assocation (n.d.). Billing and reimbursement for speech-language pathologists and audiologists. (n.d.). Retrieved November 28, 2017, from https://www.asha.org/practice/reimbursement/

Havens, L. A. (2017). Giving insurers the full treatment picture. *The ASHA Leader, 22*(4), 34–35.

International Classification of Diseases-10th Revision – Clinical Modification (n.d). Retrieved November 28, 2017, from https://www.cms.gov/Medicare/Coding/ICD10/index.html?redirect=%2FICD10

Swanson, N. (2018). New cognitive treatment code takes effect. *The ASHA Leader, 23*(1), 24–26.

CHAPTER 14

Insurance

Who

There are many types of health insurances across the country and there are many different categories of insurances. Specific insurances for certain age groups or disabilities also exist. For instance, Medicare is likely something you have heard of before as it is the federal insurance coverage for persons over age 65. But did you know that Medicare may also cover younger people with certain disabilities and people with end-stage renal disease (permanent kidney failure requiring dialysis or a transplant, sometimes called ESRD) (Medicare a, n.d.)?

There are various categories of insurance: federally funded insurance plans (Medicare and Medicaid), health maintenance organizations (HMO), preferred provider organization (PPO), and high deductible health plans (HDHP), just to name a few (American Speech-Language-Hearing Assocation, n.d.). Each insurance may have their own rules and regulations regarding services covered, how much a patient is required to pay out of pocket, referral requirements, and prior authorizations, along with a host of billing guidelines and restrictions. Most clinicians will not need to learn the specific details of all the companies, but it is always wise to have a basic understanding of the principles so you can provide the most comprehensive ethical services while getting paid for your work.

What

To further expand on the categories described above, we will start with definitions of categories and then examine how that may affect you as a clinician. As stated earlier, Medicare is a federally funded program, primarily the key insurance for persons over age 65. Medicare may also cover younger people who have certain disabilities as well as patients with end-stage renal failure. Because Medicare is federally funded, a federal entity sets pricing and coverage policies. There may be some regional differences in reimbursement rates, and from state to state there may be some differences on what services are covered. There are different subsections to Medicare. Medicare Part A covers hospital, skilled nursing facility care, hospice care, and home health care. Medicare Part B covers services from doctors, outpatient care, home health care, durable medcial equipment, and some preventative services. Medicare Part C (or Medicare Advantage) is Part A and B coverage that is provided by private insurances approved by Medicare, but may also provide additional services for the member. Medicare Part D is another portion that is managed by approved private insurances to cover prescription drug costs. For Medicare Part A, there are deductibles and coinsurance costs for the member while for Parts B, C, and D, there are additional out-of-pocket premiums that a member must pay (Medicare b, n.d.).

Medicaid primarily covers families who fall in the low-income bracket, qualifying pregnant women and children, and individuals who are receiving supplement security income (SSI)/those who qualify for disability benefits (Medicaid, n.d.). Medicaid is a combination of state and federally funded programs, which means that while there are certain rules and regulations at the federal level that will be consistent regardless of state. There are also some specific policies and coverages within each state. Examples of differences include requirements for obtaining prior authorization for services and required referral information.

Health maintenance organization (HMO) plans are entire medical communities who agree to provide services. With an HMO, you must select a primary care physician who will coordinate your health care needs by providing referrals to specialists. Preferred provider organization (PPO) plans are network plans that give a person access to any provider within the network without a specific referral from a primary care physician. PPO plans may give access to providers outside the network, but a member would need to verify that before seeking services. High deductible health plans (HDHP) cross categories as they could be HMO plans, PPO plans, or some other type of plan (eHealth Insurance, n.d.). The common theme with the HDHP plans are that they have a lower monthly premium with a higher deductible for the member.

Regardless of the type of plan a client may have, you as the clinician will need a National Provider Identifier. This is a number specific to you as the clinician (free to obtain) that is needed to bill insurance entities. You will also need to apply for provider numbers with Medicare, Medicaid, and some private insurance companies in order to bill. Depending on the setting in which you work, you may not be billing insurance companies or you may only bill certain companies, so it is not always required to have a number unless you will be billing.

When billing, keep in mind that the amount you bill will likely not be the amount that is reimbursed. Your fees should be set by considering the cost of providing the services and should only be set after lots of research and thought. As stated previously, some insurances have set rates for certain codes and it may be necessary with some companies to establish a contract with a fee schedule that both parties agree to before you bill them. There may be certain restrictions that require receiving authorization prior to providing services or you will not get reimbursed. Once you or your company determine the insurance companies you will work with, you must also remember that your fee schedule must be firm. You cannot charge various amounts for different clients based on the type of insurance or their ability to pay. You may be able to have policies in place to allow for variation, but these policies should be very specific and should only be set after seeking legal counsel or doing other research to make sure you are abiding by insurance codes and laws.

Why

Most clients are covered by some type of insurance. If you work in a medical setting, billing practices and procedures will likely already be determined for you. If you start your own private practice, you may need to set up the contracts, policies, procedures, and billing initiatives. You will always want to make sure you have permission from the client to share their information with the insurance company. Recall from Chapter 2, Referrals, the Health Insurance Portability and Accountability Act (HIPAA). This assures clients that you will not share their information with any parties other than those you have permission to do so with. This includes insurance companies as you are often required to send office notes or other information along with the client's demographic information and billing codes.

As clinicians, we want to provide the highest standard in care to our clients, which also includes billing practices. Insurance companies require a certain standard of care and are in place to make sure clients receive services as needed. In order to stay in business, clinicians will need to be reimbursed for their time and knowledge. Along with correct billing procedures, clinicians will also want to make sure their documentation of evaluation and treatment contains the required information. Some insurance companies have specific requirements regarding information contained within reports or other documentation. Requirements such as time spent with the client, the type of services provided, the skilled interventions used, and prognosis may need to be sent with billing.

When

Insurance will be billed after services are provided. Clinicians must make sure they are only billing for services that were provided and that they are providing all the required documentation to the insurance company. Correct coding initiatives must be in place and clinicians must make sure they are using the most specific codes available for ICD-10 (diagnosis codes) as well as CPT (procedure codes) codes. Clinicians should not unbundle codes. This means that if there is a code that includes all the components covered, the clinician should use the code that represents the work completed as a whole, rather than breaking down each part and billing separately for individual sections. So, if a clinician completes a speech sound inventory as well as an expressive and receptive language evaluation, the clinician should use the 92523 code which is inclusive of all those components, as opposed to billing a separate code for each of the tests given.

There may be work to be done prior to seeing the client in regards to insurance. Prior authorization may need to be obtained from the insurance company to make sure the services will be covered. If a service is not covered under the client's insurance policy, then the clinician or staff should let the client know and make sure they are aware of the costs related to receiving the services. If a client has an HMO, you will have to have the doctor's referral prior to providing the services or the procedures will not be covered. For Medicare, physician referrals are required for speech-language services, while for Medicaid, it varies from state to state.

There are many considerations when dealing with insurance companies. Many private insurance companies' policies are loosely set based on federal programs, but that does not mean they are all alike. For instance, some private insurance companies do not cover speech therapy unless the cause of the communication disorder is related to a medical diagnosis or event. In these situations, an evaluation may be covered, but if the client has a communication disorder that is not medically related, they consider it to be a developmental disorder and their definition of developmental includes being able to "grow out of it"; therefore, treatment would not be covered and would be an out-of-pocket cost to the family. Another interesting piece of information related to covered services is that Medicare has certain caps on services. This means that there are limits for how much they will cover on an annual basis. When the legislation was being passed on outpatient therapeutic services it read, "occupational therapy, physical therapy and speech therapy." Therapy amounts were set so that a certain amount was given annually for occupational therapy and that same amount was given to physical therapy and speech therapy combined, all because there was not a comma after physical therapy. So, for instance, a person covered under Medicare can receive $1,980 annually for occupational therapy, but physical therapy and speech therapy must share $1,980 between the two services. There are modifiers that can be used to extend the amount, but the point is that sometimes policies and procedures are passed by people who may not be trained in our field so clinicians cannot count on any two companies having the same coverage. A new development in 2018 is that the Medicare caps have been lifted and patients who need services are eligible without having a particular coverage limit (Washington Post, n.d.). With this change, there may still be a requirement that certain justification is presented as well as a modifier used when billing, but this should show clinicians that it is our responsibility to do our research and review insurance policies and billing procedures.

Where

Depending on your place of employment, you may or may not be directly related to billing practices. In most school systems, services are provided as part of federal/state money through Individualized Education Plans. You will want to check with the director of services for students with special needs to determine if there are billing practices you need to be aware of. In most all other settings, unless you work for an entity that receives money via other methods, you will be involved to some degree with billing. While you may not be the primary person responsible for speaking with insurance companies, you may be responsible for providing someone within the office with the information to provide to insurance companies, and you are ethically required to make sure only services you provide are billed and the highest level of coding practices are used.

How

For each person insured, there will be a subscriber number. If the policy is in the name of the patient, they are considered the primary subscriber. If the client is covered by his/her parents' insurance policy, the company will need information on the primary subscriber (parent) as well as the client's information. Billing forms should be developed based on providing the most accurate information in one place. This should include information such as the client's name, date of birth, address, subscriber number, group number (if applicable), and guarantor (person responsible for payment or the primary subscriber on the insurance). It is also important to clearly document the ICD-10 (diagnosis code) and CPT (procedure code) codes. A copy of the insurance card should also be included in the client's chart so that the office will have access to additional information, such as the contact information for the insurance company, should it be needed. If possible, it is always best to contact the insurance company prior to arrival of the client or during the initial session. Important information, such as if there is a co-pay required from the client or if services must have prior approval, can be determined and discussed with the client/family at the time of initial services.

The insurance world changes often. Staying aware and informed of changes within the nation and your state will help make sure you are not only providing the highest level of care, but also helping your company stay in business. Because of the variability among coverages, continuous training in this area will be beneficial. There are many helpful resources available to assist clinicians in learning the basics, some are provided for you in the reference section of this chapter.

Top 10 Terms

Health maintenance organization (HMO)

Preferred provider organization (PPO)

High deductible health plan (HDHP)

Medicare

Medicaid

National Provider Identifier (NPI)

Health Insurance Portability and Accountability Act (HIPAA)

Prior authorization

Individualized Education Plans

Primary care physician

Chapter Tips

1. Not all insurances are the same. Insurance coverage varies. Different companies may be available dependening on age or disability and could be private insurance or federally funded programs.

2. Most all insurance policies require referrals and prior authorization. Information should be kept on file and insurance companies should be called prior to the arrival of the client or during the first session.

3. Different insurance companies require different information to be included on documentation, and some companies require additional information to be submitted with billing documents.

Activities

14–1.

Insurance

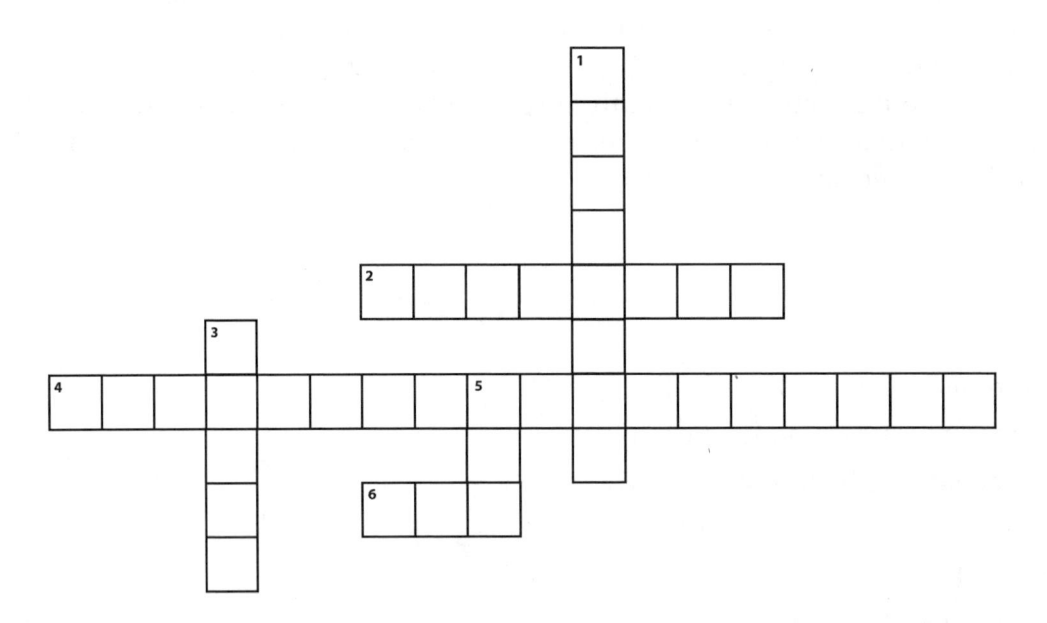

Down:
1. Federally funded program primarily for individuals over 65
3. Out of pocket expense a member must pay per visit
5. Private insurance that requires management of services by a primary care physician

Across:
2. Federally funded program primarily for low income families
4. Determining coverage eligibility and requirements for members
6. Private insurance that does not typically require referrals for specialists

Figure 14–1. Insurance crossword puzzle needed to complete Activity 14–1.

14–2. Using the model superbill in Figure 14–2, determine the client's name, date of birth, insurance carrier, subscriber ID, ICD-10 code, and CPT code.

Speech and Hearing Clinic (CHARGE CAPTURE)

Patient Full Name	Oliver C. Square	Patient DOB	01/01/2004
Patient Address	123 My Street		
City, State, Zip	Everywhere, NC 28000		
Patient Phone	123-456-1234	PROVIDER	
Referring Physician	Dr. Medical		
Insurance Carrier	Medicaid	Patient PMT$	
Insurance ID	9001004500P		
Preauthorization#			

HEARING DIAGNOSIS

H90.6 Mixed;bilateral	H90.0 Conductive hearing loss; bilateral	H93.25 Auditory Processing Dis
H90.71 mixed;unilat right	H90.11 Conductive hearing loss; right	H91.23 Sudden hearing loss
H90.72 mixed; unilat left	H90.12 Conductive hearing loss; left	H83.3x9 Noise Induced hrng loss
Z01.10 hearing screen	H90.3 Sensorineural hearing loss	F45.8 Functional hearing loss

HEARING CHARGES

Testing

92551	Pass/Fail "Screening"
92555	Speech audiometry threshold
92556	Speech audiometry threshold w/ recog
92557	Comprehensive Audiometry Threshold
92567	Tympanometry;middle ear/eardrum test
92582	Conditioned Play Audiometry
92587	Distortion emission;3-11 frequencies per ear

DEVICES/PROGRAMMING

V5011	HA fitting/orientation
V5014	Repair/Modification/Adjust
V5110	Dispensing Fee
V5253	HA;Digital; Binaural BTE
V5264	Ear mold; non-disposable
V5275	Ear impression; each

Evaluations

92626	Hearing Aid Testing(Rehab status); 60 min
92620	Eval w/ Report;Central Auditory; 60 min
92625	Tinnitus Assessment(pitch/loud/masking)

SPEECH DIAGNOSIS

F80.1 Expressive Lng. Dis	I69.990 Apraxia Following Unspec CVA	R47.0 Aphasia	F84.0 Autism
(F80.2) Mixed Exp/Rec Lgn Di	R13.14 Dysphagia	R47.1 Dysarthria	F98.5 Fluency; adulthd onset
F80.0 Phonology Dis.	I69.992 Facial Weakness following CVA	R49.2 Dysphonia	F80.81 Fluency; childhd onset

SPEECH CHARGES

Testing/Evaluation Charges

92521	Speech Fluency Eval(eg. Stuttering)
92522	Speech Sound Production(eg. Articualtion)
(92523)	Speech Sound Production w/ Language comprehension and expressive evaluation
92524	Behavioral and qualitative analysis of voice and resonance

Treatment Charges

92507	Tx of speech, lang., voice, communication and/or auditory disorder; individual
92508	Tx of speech, lang., voice, communication and/or auditory disorder; group

CATEGORY	CURRENT	GOAL	DISCHARGE	IMPAIRMENT LVL.	
Speech	G8999	G9186	G9158	CI	1-19%
Compreh.	G9159	G9160	G9161	CJ	20-39%
Expression	G9162	G9163	G9164	CK	40-59%
Voice	G9171	G9172	G9173	CL	60-79%

Figure 14–2. Example model superbill needed to complete Activity 14–2.

Answers to Activities

14–1.

Insurance

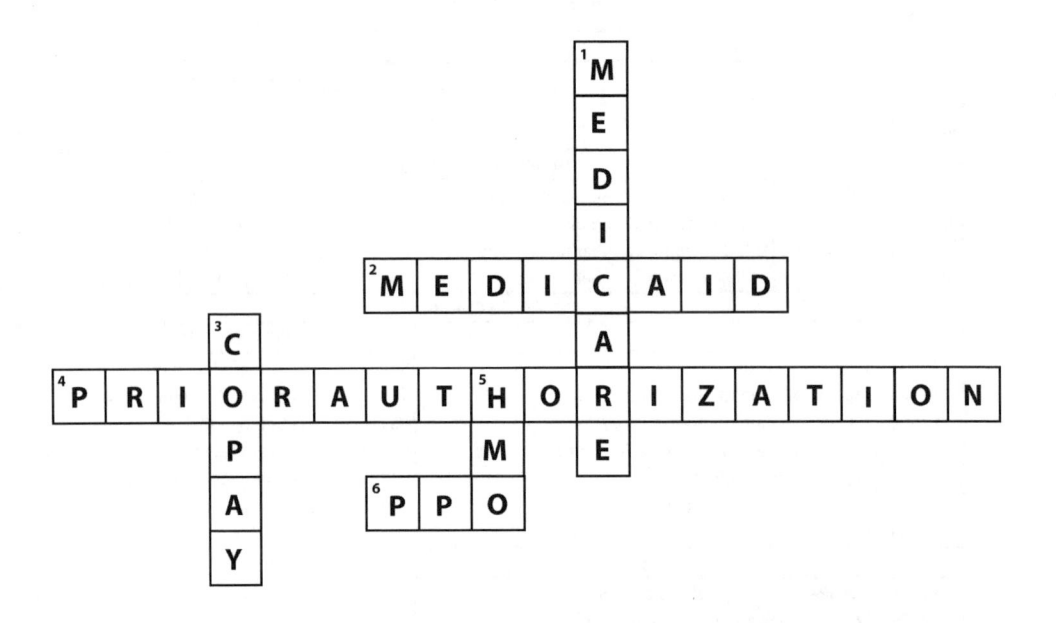

```
            ¹M
             E
             D
             I
       ²M E D I C A I D
       ³C         A
    ⁴P R I O R A U T ⁵H O R I Z A T I O N
       P         M   E
       A       ⁶P P O
       Y
```

Down:
1. Federally funded program primarily for individuals over 65
3. Out of pocket expense a member must pay per visit
5. Private insurance that requires management of services by a primary care physician

Across:
2. Federally funded program primarily for low income families
4. Determining coverage eligibility and requirements for members
6. Private insurance that does not typically require referrals for specialists

Figure 14–3. Answers to Activity 14–1.

14-2.

Speech and Hearing Clinic (CHARGE CAPTURE)			
Patient Full Name	Oliver C. Square	Patient DOB	01/01/2004
Patient Address	123 My Street		
City, State, Zip	Everywhere, NC 28000		
Patient Phone	123-456-1234	PROVIDER	
Referring Physician	Dr. Medical		
Insurance Carrier	Medicaid	Patient PMT$	
Insurance ID	9001004500P		
Preauthorization#			

NAME → (Patient Full Name) ← DOB
Insurance → (Insurance Carrier)
Subscriber ID → (Insurance ID)

HEARING DIAGNOSIS

H90.6 Mixed;bilateral	H90.0 Conductive hearing loss; bilateral	H93.25 Auditory Processing Dis
H90.71 mixed;unilat right	H90.11 Conductive hearing loss; right	H91.23 Sudden hearing loss
H90.72 mixed; unilat left	H90.12 Conductive hearing loss; left	H83.3x9 Noise Induced hrng loss
Z01.10 hearing screen	H90.3 Sensorineural hearing loss	F45.8 Functional hearing loss

HEARING CHARGES

Testing

92551	Pass/Fail "Screening"
92555	Speech audiometry threshold
92556	Speech audiometry threshold w/ recog
92557	Comprehensive Audiometry Threshold
92567	Tympanometry;middle ear/eardrum test
92582	Conditioned Play Audiometry
92587	Distortion emission;3-11 frequencies per ear

DEVICES/PROGRAMMING

V5011	HA fitting/orientation
V5014	Repair/Modification/Adjust
V5110	Dispensing Fee
V5253	HA;Digital; Binaural BTE
V5264	Ear mold; non-disposable
V5275	Ear impression; each

Evaluations

92626	Hearing Aid Testing(Rehab status); 60 min
92620	Eval w/ Report;Central Auditory; 60 min
92625	Tinnitus Assessment(pitch/loud/masking)

SPEECH DIAGNOSIS

F80.1 Expressive Lng. Dis	I69.990 Apraxia Following Unspec CVA	R47.0 Aphasia	F84.0 Autism
F80.2 Mixed Exp/Rec Lgn Di	R13.14 Dysphagia	R47.1 Dysarthria	F98.5 Fluency; adulthd onset
F80.0 Phonology Dis.	I69.992 Facial Weakness following CVA	R49.2 Dysphonia	F80.81 Fluency; childhd onset

ICD-10 ↓ (F80.2 Mixed Exp/Rec Lgn Di circled)

SPEECH CHARGES

Testing/Evaluation Charges

92521	Speech Fluency Eval(eg. Stuttering)
92522	Speech Sound Production(eg. Articualtion)
92523	Speech Sound Production w/ Language comprehension and expressive evaluation
92524	Behavioral and qualitative analysis of voice and resonance

CPT → (92523 circled)

Treatment Charges

92507	Tx of speech, lang., voice, communication and/or auditory disorder; individual
92508	Tx of speech, lang., voice, communication and/or auditory disorder; group

CATEGORY	CURRENT	GOAL	DISCHARGE	IMPAIRMENT LVL	
Speech	G8999	G9186	G9158	CI	1-19%
Compreh.	G9159	G9160	G9161	CJ	20-39%
Expression	G9162	G9163	G9164	CK	40-59%
Voice	G9171	G9172	G9173	CL	60-79%

Figure 14–4. Answers to Activity 14–2.

Wrap-Up

1. Look at your insurance card. Can you determine from your card the following information?

    Company: _____

    Subscriber ID: _____

    Group ID: _____

    Phone number to call with questions: _____

    Type of insurance? _____

    Coverage for specialty services? _____

    Do you require referrals for specialist visits? _____

    What is your co-pay? _____

2. Look online at various billing forms. Is there a particular form you like? Why do you like that form? Are there additional pieces of information you would like included on the form? If so, what information?

    _____
    _____
    _____
    _____
    _____

References

American Speech-Language-Hearing Association (n.d.). About health insurance. Retrieved November 28, 2017, from https://www.asha.org/public/coverage/

eHealth Insurance (n.d.). Different types of health insurance plans. Retrieved November 28, 2017, from https://resources.ehealthinsurance.com/individual-and-family/different-types-health-insurance-plans

Medicaid (n.d.). Eligibility. Retrieved November 28, 2017, from https://www.medicaid.gov/medicaid/eligibility/

Medicare (n.d.). What's Medicare?. Retrieved November 28, 2017, from https://www.medicare.gov/sign-up-change-plans/decide-how-to-get-medicare/whats-medicare/what-is-medicare.html

Medicare (n.d.). Your Medicare coverage choices. Retrieved November 28, 2017, from https://www.medicare.gov/sign-up-change-plans/decide-how-to-get-medicare/your-medicare-coverage-choices.html#collapse-3134

Washington Post (n.d.). Lifting therapy caps proves a load off Medicare patients' shoulders. Retrieved March 17, 2018, from https://www.washingtonpost.com/national/health-science/lifting-therapy-caps-proves-a-load-off-medicare-patients-shoulders/2018/03/14/3aaba9e2-2768-11e8-a227-fd2b009466bc_story.html?noredirect=on&utm_term=.bf25de6462dd

CHAPTER 15

Speech Sound Disorders

Who

Children who have speech sounds disorders produce errors in the phonemes that make up our language. Their errors can range from developmentally age-appropriate mistakes or dialectal variations (i.e., not considered a disorder) to unintelligible speech (i.e., considered a severe disorder). Speech sound disorders can be divided by type into the categories of articulation errors (delivery-based errors), phonological errors (language-system based), and motor speech errors (neurological-based errors). It is important to determine both the type and severity level (mild, moderate, or severe) of the speech sound disorder in order to provide effective and efficient remediation recommendations.

What

A good place to begin is a discussion of the types and severity levels common in the classification of speech sound disorders. Articulation errors are described as deletions, substitutions, distortions, or additions of the target sound. One or more articulation errors can occur in a child's speech. These errors are treated independent of one another other. The location of the error within the word (i.e., initial, medial, or final) is also identified. Thus, an example statement concerning an articulation disorder may read, "Bert, a 4-year-old male, produced /p/s/ substitutions in beginning, medial, and final position of words."

Phonological process errors are described by a variety of terms that group errors into common patterns that occur throughout the child's sound system. Example phonological processes errors include final consonant deletion, fronting, and nasal assimilation, to name only a few. For speech sound errors to be considered as phonological processes, the error pattern needs to occur across at least two phonemes and occur consistently (this is termed an active process and refers to the errors occurring in a minimum of 20% to 40% of possible occurrences depending on the system being utilized). Thus, an example statement concerning a phonological process disorder may read, "Sylvester, a 4-year-old male, produced an active process pattern of final consonant deletion on 50% of all single words tested."

Motor speech disorders are neurological disorders that are divided into childhood apraxia of speech and childhood dysarthria. Both of these disorders involve difficulty with the muscle movements needed in speech production. In apraxia of speech, the brain has difficulty programing voluntary sound productions, resulting in speech behaviors such as groping for placement, multiple inconsistent consonant errors, and increased inaccuracies as the length of words or phrases increases. Strand (2017) describes how assessing a child with a possible diagnosis of childhood apraxia of speech involves interview (medical and developmental history), observation (speech/language sample), independent speech analysis (phonetic and phonemic inventories), standard testing (receptive language), oral peripheral exam (including oral nonverbal movements), and dynamic assessment (cueing such as slowing rate of model, or visual or tactile cues). These can provide the information necessary to differentiate childhood apraxia of speech from dysarthria or a phonological speech disorder. In dysarthria, neurological impairment causes muscle weakness that can affect articulation, respiration, phonation, resonation, and prosody. The muscle weakness affects voluntary and involuntary speech production, resulting in speech behaviors such as consistent distortions and omissions of consonants and neutralizing of vowels. The error sounds that occur in motor speech disorders may be reported using articulation or phonological process terminology. Phonological process terminology is often used in describing apraxia errors, while articulatory terms are common when describing dysarthria speech errors. Speech sound characteristics are only one aspect essential in the description of apraxia or one of the various kinds of dysarthria. Prosody, respiration, phonation, and resonation must all be assessed.

A designation of a mild, moderate, or severe speech sound disorder is a judgment rating a clinician identifies. When making this designation, the clinician should take a holistic view of all the information gathered on the speech sound problem. Some standardized tests or procedures will provide guidelines to help the clinician reach this judgment. The severity level designation will be a primary factor in the intensity of treatment recommendation. The more severe the problem, the more likely treatment will be recommended for more times per week and/or more time per session.

Why

Concern for a speech sound disorder is a frequent reason for referral for evaluation to a speech-language pathologist. The American Speech-Language-Hearing Association's website noted: "The most widely cited summary of speech sound disorder prevalence is a systematic review conducted by Law, Boyle, Harris, Harkness, and Nye (2000). They reported prevalence estimates ranging from 2% to 25% of children ages 5 to 7 years" (American Speech-Language-Hearing Association, n.d.). Speech sound disorders can comprise a large portion of the clinician's case load.

When

When the client is young and has a limited ability to perform structured tests or tasks, an independent analysis of the speech behavior may be used. In an independent analysis, a description of the child's system is developed from a sample of speech. This is different from the relational analysis approach in which a comparison of the child's production is made to the adult production (Bleile, 1991; Stoel-Gammon & Dunn, 1985). An independent analysis could include a listing of the child's phonetic inventory (all the consonant sounds produced throughout his/her speech sample, e.g., /p,b,d,t,m/), a phonotactic inventory (the syllable structure produced throughout his/her speech sample, e.g., consonant-vowel [CV], consonant-vowel-consonant [CVC], vowel-consonant [VC]), and/or an identification of strategies used (preference for a phoneme or approach to developing their sound system, e.g., tetism—preference for a /t/ phoneme in many words produced or a syllable reduplication strategy for making two-syllable words such as /titi/ for sister). An independent analysis is not about identifying errors but rather describing the system the child is using.

When the child is able to participate in standardized tests, a relational analysis is usually performed with a speech sample and dynamic assessment supplementing the test results. A relational analysis compares the sounds the child produces to the way the adult produces the sound. Sounds are identified as correct if they match the adult model and in error when they are different from how the adult produces the sound. The relational analyses will be further explored in the How section.

Where

The majority of the assessment of speech sound disorders is done in the controlled environment of the testing or treatment room. Listening for how sounds are produced and then transcribing the production is a difficult task. A quiet environment can improve the accuracy of phoneme transcription. Watching the production, instead of looking down at the record form, can also be a valuable strategy when assessing speech sound production.

How

Gathering of information about the speech sound disorder in a relational analysis can take many forms. Four commonly used methods are standardized tests, stimulability testing, speech samples, and intelligibility measures. Note that a speech sound evaluation will also include an oral-facial examination containing a diadochokinetic rate, a hearing screening, and a language screening.

Single word pictures with focus sounds identified are the common stimuli used in many standardized speech sound tests. For example, the clinician shows the client a picture of a dog and asks him/her to name the picture. The clinician records on the test record form the correctness of the target phoneme(s) (e.g., in the example "dog," /d/ and /g/). The results are then organized within the form by independent sounds in articulation tests or by patterns in phonological process tests, or in some tests by both independent sounds and phonological processes. Results are compared to the normative sample of same-age peers. Many tests also include a section where the sounds are evaluated in sentences.

Stimulability testing is included in some standardized tests. In stimulability testing, a form of dynamic assessment, the clinician cues (stimulates) the client to produce the phonemes that were in error on the test. Even when not a component of the standardized test, stimulability testing of error phonemes can provide information useful in deciding severity and/or recommended goals and objectives. A direction such as, "Watch and listen, look at me and say /dʌ/" would be common in stimulability testing. The clinician may increase the length of the target from syllable (/dʌ/) to word (dog) to phrase (big dog) to sentence (I see the big dog). Cues may also be varied to determine what error sounds are most or least stimulable for the particular client. It is interesting to note that in some instances clinicians will select sounds for which the client is easily cued to recommend early treatment, perhaps increasing the likelihood that they will be successful in early therapy; while other times a stimulable sound may be monitored instead of treated with an eye for self-improvement without treatment at the same time recommending nonstimulable sounds for therapeutic intervention, perhaps because they would not likely improve without remediation.

Speech samples allow for consideration of speech sounds in a broader context than the single word or sentence format used in most standardized tests. The clinician wants a large enough sample of the client speaking so that it is representative of the client's typical speech performance. The clinician looks to see if the error sounds in the speech sample are consistent with the errors on the standardized test. The clinician can also observe the effects of rate of speech, resonance, loudness, pitch, and utterance length on the understandability of the speech produced as a whole. Clinicians have been known to lament the fact that a child can produce the phonemes correctly in the speech room but not in their conversations outside of therapy. Taking a speech sample outside the treatment room with a partner other than the clinician is recommended prior to dismissal from speech sound remediation.

The understandability of speech is termed speech intelligibility. Sometimes an estimate of the clinician's impression of intelligibility is given in a report. The problem with such an estimate is that speech intelligibility is related in part to one's experience interacting with an individual and interpreting their unique speech system. Care should be taken so that the perception of improved intelligibility is not the result of the clinician interpreting better and not the child's producing better speech. The Percentage of Consonants Correct (PCC) metric was developed by Shriberg and Kwiatkowski (1982) as a measure comparing consonants produced correctly to total consonants possible from a speech sample following prescribed rules. The PCC could be used to provide a severity rating that was not dependent on the clinician's estimate of intelligibility. The original study suggested a score of >90% = mild, 65% to 85% = mild-moderate, 50% to 65% = moderate-severe, and <50% = severe. Shriberg, Austin, Lewis, McSweeny, and Wilson (1997) provided extensions and reliability data on PCC and nine other speech sound metrics.

Top 10 Terms

Articulation disorder

Independent analysis

Intelligibility

Motor speech disorder

Percentage consonant correct metric

Phonetic inventory
Phonotactic inventory
Phonological process disorder
Relational analysis
Stimulability testing

Chapter Tips

1. Tape recording the standardized testing, stimulability testing, and conversational sample is a good idea. However, even a high-quality tape does not replace the need to record the phoneme substitutions, additions, distortions, and omissions on the recording form as they happen, but it can be useful for checking back if a question occurs. The clinician must also be cognizant not to violate HIPPA regulations when taping a speech sample.

2. Recording articulation substitutions and additions requires the use of the International Phonetic Alphabet system. Diacritic marks are useful in communication of distortion errors. Phonological processes or patterns often involve characteristics of place, manner, and voicing of the phonemes. Thus, reviewing phonetic classification and transcription will aid in your ability to assess and communicate accurately about speech sound disorders.

Activities

15–1. Identify whether each item is more closely associated with a child who most likely has an articulation disorder, phonological process disorder, or motor speech disorder by putting the appropriate term before each descriptive statement.

1. _____ Lateral lisp
2. _____ Seems language based, affects her reading too
3. _____ Produces the sound different every time he says the word
4. _____ He has this funny habit of never starting or ending a word with a vowel; he adds the /h/ sound before or after the vowel of these words
5. _____ The sound errors seem related to his cleft palate
6. _____ He has a "bad" /r/
7. _____ Her speech errors are the result of cerebral palsy
8. _____ All his errors involve the back sounds being made more forward in the mouth

15–2. There is no one universally accepted age of speech sound acquisition data. Shriberg (1993) separated the 24 consonant phonemes into the early eight: approximate ages 1 to 3; the middle eight: approximate ages 3 to 6.5; and late eight: approximate ages 5 to 7.5 In the following samples, place a 1 before the set that represents the early eight, a 2 for the middle eight, and a 3 for the late eight.

___ /ʃ/ /s/ /ð/ /θ/ /r/ /z/ /l/ /ʒ/
___ /m/ /b/ /j/ /n/ /w/ /d/ /p/ /h/
___ /t/ /ŋ/ /k/ /g/ /f/ /v/ /tʃ/ /dʒ/

15–3. Complete Table 15–1. Column 1 lists some common phonological processes. Apply that process to the word in column 2 and write how the child produced the word under the word provided.

Table 15–1. Phonological Process Name and Example

	Process Name	Example: Fill in the Word Produced When Process Applied
1	Deaffrication	/dʒʌdʒə/
2	Initial consonant voicing	/pɑp/
3	Consonant harmony or assimilation	/ɪnk/
4	Velar fronting	/sʌŋ/
5	Syllable reduction	/hɑtdɔg/
6	Final devoicing	/dɔg/
7	Stopping of fricative or velar	/ʃip/
8	Stridency deletion	/ʃip/
9	Consonant simplification	/stɑp/
10	Palatal fronting	/fit/
11	Final consonant deletion	/hæt/
12	Liquid simplification	/lɪdəl/
13	Glottal replacement	/bɑtəl/
14	Backing to velar or /h/	/tɑp/
15	Initial consonant deletion	/sɛf/

The following are some phoneme classification reminders:

Obstruent = /p,b,f,v,s,z,ʃ,ʒ,ð,θ,t,d,k,g,tʃ,dʒ/
Glide = /j,w/
Nasals = /m,n,ŋ/
Liquid = /l,r/
Strident = /f,v,s,z,ʃ,ʒ,tʃ,dʒ/
Velar = /k,g,ŋ/
Fricative = /f,v,s,z,ʃ,ʒ,ð,θ/
Affricate = /tʃ,dʒ/
Sonorant = nasals, liquids, and glides
Glottal stop = ʔ

Answers to Activities

15–1.

1. Articulation disorder
2. Phonological disorder
3. Apraxia
4. Phonological disorder
5. Articulation disorder
6. Articulation disorder
7. Dysarthria
8. Phonological disorder

15–2.

_3_ /ʃ/ /s/ /ð/ /θ/ /r/ /z/ /l/ /ʒ/
_1_ /m/ /b/ /j/ /n/ /w/ /d/ /p/ /h/
_2_ /t/ /ŋ/ /k/ /g/ /f/ /v/ /tʃ/ /dʒ/

15–3. See Table 15–2. *Note*: answers are given in bold type. There are multiple correct answers for column 3.

Table 15–2. Phonological Process Example Answer Chart

	Process Name	Example: Fill in the Word Produced When Process Applied
1	Deaffrication	/dʒʌdʒə/ /fʌfə/
2	Initial consonant voicing	/pɑp/ /bɑp/
3	Consonant harmony or assimilation	/ɪnk/ /ɪŋk/
4	Velar fronting	/sʌŋ/ /sʌn/
5	Syllable reduction	/hɑtdɔg/ /dɔg/
6	Final devoicing	/dɔg/ /dɔk/
7	Stopping of fricative or velar	/ʃip/ /tip/
8	Stridency deletion	/ʃip/ /tip/
9	Consonant simplification	/stɑp/ /tɑp/
10	Palatal fronting	/fit/ /mit/
11	Final consonant deletion	/hæt/ /hæ/
12	Liquid simplification	/lɪdəl/ /wɪdəl/
13	Glottal replacement	/bɑtəl/ /bɑʔəl/
14	Backing to velar or /h/	/tɑp/ /tɑh/
15	Initial consonant deletion	/sef/ /ef/

Wrap-Up

1. Scenario: You have just begun your first job in the public school system. A teacher notes that Mr. Cross, your predecessor who has recently been promoted to clinical supervisor in your system, primarily talked about assessment of articulation disorders. She asks you to compare and contrast assessment procedures for articulation and phonological disorders. Compare and contrast articulation and phonological process assessment in the space provided—be clear, define ideas, and keep jargon to a minimum. How you provide your information is equally important to what information you provide.

2. Should you use phonetic transcription of the sounds in a report? How could you clarify the phonetic symbols for a nonspeech clinician?

3. Some standardized tests give clinicians the option of marking correct/incorrect instead of elaborating on the type of error produced. Why might a clinician choose to go beyond the simple correct/incorrect scoring?

4. Identify a word that is produced differently in your regional dialect than in another regional dialect. Which production is wrong? Why?

References

American Speech-Language-Hearing Association. (n.d.) Speech sound disorders: Articulation and phonology: Incidence and prevalence. Retrieved February 22, 2018, from http://www.asha.org/PRPSpecificTopic.aspx?folderid=8589935321§ion=Incidence_and_Prevalence

Bleile, K. M. (1991). *Child phonology: A book of exercises for students*. San Diego, CA: Singular Publishing.

Shriberg, L. (1993). Four new speech and voice-prosody measures for genetics research and other studies in developmental phonological disorders. *Journal of Speech, Language, and Hearing Research, 36*, 105–140.

Shriberg, L. D, Austin, D., Lewis, B. A. McSweeny, J. L., & Wilson, D. L. (1997). The percentage of consonants correct (PCC) metric: Extensions and reliability data. *Journal of Speech, Language & Hearing Research, 40*(4), 708–722.

Shriberg, L. D., & Kwiatkowski, J. (1982). Phonological disorders III: A procedure for assessing severity of involvement. *Journal of Speech and Hearing Disorders, 47*, 256–270.

Stoel-Gammon, C., & Dunn, C. (1985). *Normal and disordered phonology in children*. Baltimore, MD: University Park Press.

Strand, E. (2017). Appraising apraxia. *The ASHA Journal, 22*(3), 50–58.

CHAPTER 16

Voice Assessment

Who

Speech-language pathologists (SLPs) work closely with physicians, such as ear, nose, and throat physicians or otolaryngologists, to evaluate and treat voice and resonance disorders. Voice disorders are typically differences of loudness, pitch, and/or quality that differ from the established norms for age, gender, geographic location, or cultural background (Aronson & Bless, 2009; Boone, McFarlane, Von Berg, & Zarik, 2014). A patient could present with vocal problems at any age.

A physician, ideally one who specializes in voice such as an otolaryngologist, will provide medical clearance for patients. When completing an evaluation for a voice problem, the clinician must have a referral from a physician who specializes in voice prior to the evaluation. In some instances, a clinician may be conducting an evaluation and the clinician notices a potential voice problem; in that case, the clinician must refer the patient to the physician to receive medical clearance prior to starting therapy.

What

This workbook has discussed various speech and language disorders. Voice is under the broad umbrella of speech; therefore, problems with voice indicate that a patient would have a speech disorder. Evaluation requires specialized knowledge of articulatory, phonatory, and respiratory anatomy and physiology as well as skill in instrumental assessments (Golper, 2010). Voice disorders are classified based on the cause (etiology) or symptoms (Shipley & McAffe, 2016). Etiology for voice disorders can be considered as either organic (having a physiological change that has occurred to cause the problem) or functional (repeated use). Voice disorders can also be psychogenic in nature, meaning the cause can be due to psychological stress. Etiology is not necessarily mutually exclusive. This means you could have a client with a voice disorder that resulted from misuse causing a physiological change. For example, a person who consistently speaks extremely loudly may cause vocal nodules to develop; their functional misuse causes a physiological change in the vocal fold tissue. For the purposes of the book, we will focus on organic and functional causes. Clinicians should keep in mind that in the instances of psychogenic causes a referral to the appropriate professional should be made.

Why

Voice evaluations are important for helping a patient know and/or learn how to use their voice appropriately in order to help keep a functional problem from developing into a physiological change. They are also useful in helping a patient know what can be expected for their voice function based on their physiological status. A patient who has a paralyzed vocal fold may need different techniques for voicing and to keep them from harming themselves trying to vocalize sounds. Functional goals are often recommended for voice patients. These types of goals are determined based on what the patient identifies as being important to them. A comprehensive voice assessment will help determine the feasibility of the goals the patient is hoping to pursue.

When

A screening may be a starting point for a patient. Vocal screenings can be done quickly by the clinician talking with the patient and paying close attention to the patient's resonance, pitch, loudness, and vocal quality (American Speech-Language-Hearing Association, n.d.). If a screening is determined to be within normal limits, a complete evaluation may not be warranted.

If a patient were to present with concerns over their voice, a clinician were to perceive vocal differences that should be explored, or a patient is referred by a physician for vocal concerns, then a more formal voice evaluation should be completed.

Where

Voice screening or evaluations can be done in a typical clinical setting. Particular attention should be given to the amount of background noise in the area where a voice evaluation will occur to make sure the clinician will not have any difficulty hearing potential slight changes in a patient's voice during testing. If equipment will be used during the evaluation, the area should be checked for adequate electrical access. Most equipment used in a voice evaluation will be either on a desktop computer, laptop, or cart where the equipment stays.

How

Comprehensive assessment for voice disorders will include a variety of areas. Case history will again play a vital role in the assessment process and can help determine vocal habits. Self-assessment questionnaires can also be very helpful in a voice evaluation to determine how the patient perceives their voice, identifying vocal behaviors they may be using, as well as onset of symptoms and a timeline of when the symptoms began. Oral-peripheral examinations are important in a voice evaluation. A clinician should determine there are no physical abnormalities in the oral cavity, or document what abnormalities are present, as well as check for symmetry, strength, range of motion, and sensation. More information can be found in Chapter 4, Oral-Facial Examinations.

A clinician will want to document the respiratory abilities of the patient. Respiratory patterns, such as unusual breathing (e.g., clavicular breathing), speaking during inhalation, taking excessive breaths, or running out of breath when using short sentences/phrases, should be documented. An s/z ratio is an effective task that can help determine respiratory and phonatory efficiency (Prater, Swift, Deem, & Miller, 2000). This is done by having the patient sustain each of the phonemes (s/z) while the clinician keeps track of time for each. The ratio is determined and can be compared to norms for age. Ratios within normal limits and sustained for the amount of time expected for age indicate normal respiratory ability and no vocal pathology, while ratios within the norm with less duration indicate a respiratory problem, and ratios not within the norm (but with normal or above time sustained) could be indicative of a laryngeal pathology.

When assessing for vocal problems, the clinician will need to keep in mind some physics terms. Frequency is the number of completed cycles that occur in 1-sec time. As clinicians, we think of frequency in terms of pitch of voice. Vocal folds that open at a rate of 220 cycles per second would have a frequency of 220 hertz (Hz) and would have a higher perceived pitch than a person who has a vocal frequency of 180 Hz. Loudness is measured in decibels (dB). A person who speaks with loudness of 55 dB would be perceived as a louder speaker than a person who speaks at 40 dB.

It is also important to use quality descriptors when assessing for voice. Terms such as harsh (hoarse or coarse), shrill (too high pitch), scratchy, and rough (sounds gravelly) may be terms the clinician uses to describe the patient's vocal quality. Pitch, loudness, and quality are areas that are typically considered grouped together when assessing voice. A clinician can use a variety of methods to assess these areas including self-checklists, having the patient repeat phrases or sentences, formal assessment tools (which give a systematic way to describe and quantify vocal abilities), or even using some instrumentation to formally evaluate the frequency and loudness of their voice.

Resonance is another area that should be assessed during a voice evaluation. Resonance is the amount of air that passes through the nasal passages while a person is speaking. As clinicians, you should be familiar with the sounds and characteristics of sounds including the nasal sounds (a review can be found in Chapter 4). Sounds such as /m/ and /n/ are considered nasals and should be produced with some nasal quality; however, not all sounds should have that nasal quality. A patient could be determined to be hypernasal (too much air passing through the nasal cavity), hyponasal (too little air passing through the nasal cavity), normal, or with cul-de-sac resonance (when sound is resonated in the throat but gets stuck there resulting in the patient sounding muffled) (Speech Language Therapy Info, n.d.).

Assessing phonation and rate are also part of the evaluation process. A clinician will need to asses a patient's ability to sustain a sound consistently and for a given period of time based on norms for age and gender. Quality terms may be used often in this part of the examination. Rate of voice onset/offset as well as overall speech rate will also need to be assessed.

Many instrumental options are available for assisting in the voice evaluation. Instruments may be available in all areas of the voice evaluation. There are too many options available to cover for this workbook; however, some frequently used instruments are mentioned here. For laryngoscopic examinations, a clinician may use an oral mirror to obtain a visual of the vocal tract and vocal fold closure; a flexible endoscope (a tube that is flexible and has a camera/light on the end) to determine the integrity of the nasal or oral cavity, larynx, and vocal folds; or stroboscopy (a tube with a camera and light that can take video/pictures), which is more helpful in visualizing the vocal folds as they open and close as it takes images and allows the clinician to view the functioning of the vocal folds in what seems like slow motion. For acoustic analysis, one piece of equipment on the market is the Computerized Speech Lab, which allows the clinician to obtain data on fundamental frequency, habitual pitch, maximum phonation time, among others. While using computerized equipment is not vital in an assessment, it is very helpful to get specific data as well as provide a visual representation of a patient's voice. PRAAT is a computer program that can be useful for visualizing vocal patterns as well as determining differences in jitter (pitch differences of the voice) or shimmer (amplitude differences of the voice).

Top 10 Terms

Etiology

Organic disorders

Functional disorders

Frequency

Amplitude

Resonance

Phonation

Respiration

Jitter

Shimmer

Chapter Tips

1. Medical clearance is extremely important when working with patients who are exhibiting voice problems. Ideally, the patient will come to the evaluation appointment with medical clearance; however, if they do not and a vocal problem is identified, you must refer the patient to a physician to be evaluated.

2. Voice problems are not exclusive. They can occur as a combination of organic, functional, or psychogenic problems. Determining the etiology will assist in developing appropriate goals to ensure safety and functionality of the patient's voice.

3. Many areas should be evaluated when assessing for voice disorders. Respiratory, acoustic analysis, vocal habits, and resonance are all areas that should be addressed.

Activities

16–1. Match the following quality terms to the patients described in the following sentences:

A. Harsh
B. Breathy
C. Shrill
D. Raspy
E. Quiet

_____ The patient does not use a lot of voiced sounds; rather, sounds are produced with additional air.

_____ It is uncomfortable to listen to this person talking. The patient sounds mad or angry when speaking; you can almost visualize their vocal folds slamming together as they talk.

_____ The patient talks in a high-pitched voice that seems strained.

_____ It is difficult to hear this patient talking. You continuously have to keep asking them to repeat what they said.

_____ The patient's voice seems to come and go. The patient continuously clears his/her throat. After the clearing, the voice is a bit stronger for a few words then it seems to go out again.

16–2. Read the following descriptions of patients and determine if the etiology is likely organic (O), functional (F), or a combination (C).

_____ A 96-year-old female with severe osteoporosis whose torso is constantly bent forward. Her sentences sound very choppy and she cannot seem to say more than three or four words without taking additional breaths.

_____ A 35-year-old male who recently had surgery. He reported no problems prior to his surgery, but after his surgery he can only make a true voiced sound occasionally. He cannot sustain /a/ at all.

_____ A 15-year-old female who describes her voice as harsh. She was a cheerleader in middle-school and started noticing her voice stopped sounding clear. She reported that although it did not feel good, she continued to cheer and force her voice to be loud approximately 3 to 4 hr per day. The report from the otolaryngologist revealed vocal nodules through a flexible endoscopy.

_____ A 22-year-old male presents with a scratchy voice. He is a teacher who reports having laryngitis at least once every 6 weeks. He missed so much work the first half of the school year that he cannot take anymore sick leave, so he no longer takes off work when he gets laryngitis.

Answers to Activities

16–1.
B
A
C
E
D

16–2.
O
O
C
F

Wrap-Up

1. Look at the American Speech-Language-Hearing Association's (ASHA) scope of practice for SLPs. What is the position statement for the use of endoscopy, by an SLP, in assessing voice? Follow up by looking at the licensing board of the state in which you would like to practice—do they have any special stipulations or wording in their licensing laws regarding the use of endoscopy or other instrumentation used in voice assessments? Write down the gist of the ASHA statement as well as the licensing law for your state.

   ASHA:
   _____
   _____
   _____
   _____
   _____
   _____
   _____

State:

_____
_____
_____
_____
_____
_____

2. Look online at three different vocal quality or vocal behavior checklists. Choose 15 behaviors you would include if you were developing your own checklist? What kind of rating scale would you use?

   1. _____
   2. _____
   3. _____
   4. _____
   5. _____
   6. _____
   7. _____
   8. _____
   9. _____
   10. _____
   11. _____
   12. _____
   13. _____
   14. _____
   15. _____

Rating Scale:

_____
_____
_____
_____

References

American Speech-Language-Hearing Association (n.d.). Voice assessment. Retrieved January 13, 2018, from http://www.asha.org/PRP SpecificTopic.aspx?folderid=8589942600&section=Assessment

Aronson, A. E., & Bless, D. M. (2009). *Clinical voice disorders*. New York, NY: Thieme Medical Publishers.

Boone, D. R., & McFarlane, S. C. (2014). *The voice and voice therapy*. Boston: Allyn and Bacon.

Golper, L. A. (2010). *Medical speech-language pathology: A desk reference* (3rd ed.). Clifton Park, NY: Delmar.

Prater, R.J, Swift, R.W., Deem, J.F., & Miller, L (2000). *Manual of voice therapy* (2nd ed.). Austin, TX: Pro-Ed.

Shipley, K. G., & McAfee, J. G. (2016). *Assessment in speech-language pathology* (5th ed.). Boston, MA: Cengage Learning.

Speech Language Therapy Info (n.d.) Voice. Retrieved January 13, 2018, from https://www.sltinfo.com/instrumental-measurement-of-voice/

CHAPTER 17

Fluency Assessment

Who

Fluency is the flow of speech. Patients who have difficulty with a smooth flow of speech may be exhibiting a fluency disorder. Fluency disorders is a larger term that describes either stuttering (hesitant speech, interjections, use of part or whole word repetitions, or prolongations) or cluttering (rapid speech, dysrhythmic speech, unorganized thoughts/words, and often unintelligible speech). Fluency disorders are involuntary, meaning the patient does not willingly have these disfluencies in their flow of speech.

Everyone occasionally exhibits some disfluencies, like interjections of words. While disfluent speech can begin at any age, we most often see the development of disfluency in children. There are typical developmental patterns, such as a time when a preschooler may exhibit stuttering behaviors, that are considered normal. A difficult aspect of the assessment process is to determine if a preschooler who is disfluent is exhibiting typically developing disfluencies, stuttering, or cluttering.

What

There are many different aspects to consider when assessing for a fluency disorder. The clinician must determine if the disfluencies are normal disfluencies (as everyone experiences some disfluency) or a disorder. Things like interjections (e.g., "um") and revisions are often considered normal disfluencies. Whole-word repetitions, sound prolongations, and blocks may be associated with a fluency disorder or stuttering. Patients who stutter may develop secondary behaviors that are thought to occur in response to or in anticipation of the disfluency. If these secondary behaviors lead to the speaker having some success in being able to maneuver through the disfluency, they may become habitual. Secondary behaviors could be things like eye blinks, movement of the head in a particular way, tapping or snapping fingers, or pursing the lips.

Preschoolers often exhibit a period of time when their speech is more disfluent. These normal disfluencies may be alarming to parents and others involved in the child's life; however, oftentimes the child who experiences disfluencies during this stage would not be considered to have a disorder.

Multicultural issues must also be considered when determining the appropriate steps to complete an evaluation. While a clinician is not expected to be skilled in knowing all the various aspects surrounding every culture, it is recommended that some research and thought be put into the plan for evaluation prior to seeing the patient. As Robinson and Crow point out, it is important for clinicians to be mindful of cultural attributes of communication styles and expectations, myths related to etiological factors, and modifications that may need to be made to the evaluation process to be sensitive to cultural differences (1998).

Cluttering is primarily categorized as a rapid speech rate. Patients who clutter often exhibit other behaviors such as excessive disfluencies (those that are not typically categorized as normal disfluencies), monotone voice, sound distortions and omissions, and a lack of awareness of the speech disorder (Shipley & McAfee, 2016). A person who clutters may also have a language disorder combined with the disfluent speech.

Why

Stuttering disorders can be very emotionally draining for a patient. There are many emotions that may be felt by the patient and the clinician plays a vital role in helping a patient improve their communication skills and outlook. The patient may experience high levels of stress when communicating. Determining what strategies could be used help relieve some of the communication tension can lead to a much improved life for the patient.

Patients who experience cluttering may not realize that they are having difficulty communicating. They may see that people have a hard time communicating with them, but they often attribute it to someone else having the problem, not them. The evaluation process may help the patient identify some issues within their speech patterns that are causing problems with others understanding them.

When

Disfluencies may occur at any stage of life, although we often see the initial evidence of a true disfluency disorder after the stage of typically developing disfluency. There is adult-onset disfluency, but it is not as common as fluency problems that develop during childhood. Whereas stuttering is often diagnosed in children, cluttering is not usually diagnosed until a patient is an adult. One theory of the later diagnosis of cluttering is the patient's lack of awareness of their fluency problem(s).

Where

Disfluent speech can occur in any situation. With stuttering, one would typically see speech becoming more disfluent in situations where there is high stress (e.g., new situations/communication partners and in rushed communication exchanges). Cluttering is typically less pronounced when the patient is focusing or concentrating on their speech patterns or with strangers.

While the evaluation for fluency will most likely occur in a clinic setting or in a one-on-one situation, it is important to attempt to gather speech samples from various settings (more on this in the next section). Because fluency problems may change dramatically from setting to setting, the clinician cannot assume that what they find in the clinical setting is what the patient experiences across the board.

How

Case histories are extremely important when assessing for a fluency disorder. Because stuttering can cause feelings of anger, frustration, and rejection, gathering a thorough case history from the patient (or caregiver) can help determine onset time and avoidance behaviors. With patients who clutter, the clinician may find that the patient has a lack of awareness of the disorder and may only be there at the prompting of someone else. Checklists may also be very helpful in the assessment process. Checklists can help patients determine situations and feelings that may be present. The clinician can also use checklists to help guide treatment and track changes over time.

Speech samples may be one of the most important aspects of a fluency evaluation. Speech samples should be collected from more than one setting and situation. In order to get a more complete picture of the fluency problems a patient may be experiencing, speech samples should be obtained when speech is the most fluent, least fluent, and with typical disfluencies, as well as from a variety of speaking situations. With technology options today, it is easier to get these samples. A clinician could have a patient (or caregiver) record speech samples and share those with the clinician for review. If using this method, the clinician will want to make sure they have a conversation with the patient or caregiver so that instructions are clear and the clinician understands the representative nature of the sample(s). The clinician will also want to make sure they are following the policies of their workplace regarding safeguarding protected health information through HIPAA regulations (Centers for Medicare & Medicaid Services, n.d.).

After obtaining the speech sample, the clinician will need to conduct some analyses and calculations. Determining the disfluency index is one way to analyze a speech sample. The disfluency index is done to determine the percentage of disfluent speech present in a speech sample. There are several different methods for this analysis. Some clinicians will analyze the speech sample by transcribing the sample as well as the disfluencies. An example of this would be if a patient said, "Sh-Sh-Sh-She went to the store": they would transcribe this as "(PW3) She went to the store." This would indicate that the patient had three part-word repetitions of "she" before producing "She went to the store." They would continue to use this method for all disfluencies in the speech sample. The clinician would then have a chart they could refer to so that they could see all the various types of disfluencies and how often they occurred in the speech sample. Another method would be to count the disfluencies and the total number of words in that particular sample. When using this method, the clinician would count each repetition of a sound, part of a word, whole word, or phrase only once (Shipley & McAfee, 2016). For example "we-went, we-went, we-went, we-went to the movies" would count as one disfluency and five words. The total disfluency index would calculate all the disfluencies by the patient. In a 100-word phrase, if there were 10 pauses, 5 whole word repetitions, and 10 prolongations, the clinician would divide the total disfluencies by the total number of words and multiply by 100. In the above sample it would be 25 / 100 = .25 × 100 = 25% disfluencies. The clinician can calculate the total disfluencies as well as each of the individual fluency types. Using the above example if a clinician wanted to determine the percentage of the prolongations, they would divide 10 by 100 = .10 × 100 = 10% prolongations. Any of the disfluencies can be determined using the above method. Another method would be the disfluency type based on the total disfluency index. For this calculation, the clinician would divide the number of occurrences of the particular disfluency type by the total number of disfluencies and change that number to a percentage (by multiplying by 100) in order to calculate the percentage of the specific type of disfluency out of the total disfluencies. Using the above example, to determine how many of the total disfluencies were repetitions, the clinician would divide 5 (total number of repetitions) by 25 (total number of disfluencies) = .2 ×100 (to convert to a percentage) = 20% (the total percentage of repetitions). A total disfluency index of 10% or greater is typically considered to be in the disordered range (Shipley & McAfee, 2016).

Another calculation that can be done is the speech rate. This is not used solely when assessing fluency, but it can be used to assist with fluency assessments. Using the speech sample, the clinician would count the number of words produced in a particular amount of time. For example, in a 2-min sample, the clinician would count the number of words produced and divide by 2 (because the clinician is trying to determine the words per minute). If a client produced 100 words in a 30-sec interval, their speech rate would be 200 words per minute (100 words × 2, because the time sample was only 30 sec). The clinician could also calculate the overall rate including disfluencies.

Another important aspect of a fluency evaluation is determining how the speaker feels about their disfluency. The clinician will need to address this aspect in treatment and being able to evaluate the stuttering disorder from the perspective of the client is very important. One tool that could be used is a tool called OASES, which stands for the Overall Assessment of the Speaker's Experience of Stuttering (Yaruss & Quesal, 2008). Using self-checks allows the clinician to obtain information that a patient may not readily report.

When assessing for cluttering, the clinician will want to make sure they are using a comprehensive assessment model, which includes speech samples, articulation testing, and language testing. As mentioned previously, case history is very important with this population. Evaluating rate of speech (as discussed in the last paragraph) would also be vital during this assessment.

The clinician's professional judgment is vital when assessing for fluency disorders. Because there is a lack of standardized testing methods for fluency and there are multiple factors that come into play when determining if there is a fluency disorder, the clinician may need to use multiple methods and resources.

Top 10 Terms

Stuttering

Cluttering

Whole-word repetitions

Part-word repetitions

Prolongations

Disfluency index

Speech rate

Secondary characteristics

Speech sample

Normal developmental disfluency

Chapter Tips

1. Fluency is the flow of speech. Difficulties with the flow of speech may be caused by stuttering, cluttering, or a combination of both.
2. Case history and speech samples are very important when conducting a fluency evaluation.
3. Calculations such as total disfluency index and speech rate need to be understood by clinicians as these will help determine if there is a disfluency disorder present.

Activities

17-1. Using the following speech sample, determine the answers to the following questions.

"I-I-I-I really like go.....ing to school. Um I get to s-s-see my friends and it keep.......s me from being at home all the time. I enjoy be.....ing able to learn s-s-s-something new every day. My-My-My favorite part about school is s.....eeing my friends. The worst part of s......chool is the endless hours of homework."

_____ **1.** Total number of words

_____ **2.** Total number of prolongations

_____ **3.** Total number of part-word repetitions

_____ **4.** Total number of whole-word repetitions

_____ **5.** Total number of interjections

_____ **6.** Total disfluency index

_____ **7.** Total part-word repetition index

17-2. Using the following speech sample, make the following calculations.

"I l......ook forward to summer va-va-va-vacation all year long. I.......t is the bes......t part-part-part of the year, we don't ha......ve to go to s-s-s-school and we can-can-can just have...... fun all the time. We do n-n-n-not have a worry in the w........orld. Summer is n......ever long enough."

_____ **1.** Words per minute if the above sample occurred in 30 sec.
_____ **2.** Words per minute if the above sample occurred in 20 sec.
_____ **3.** Words per minute if the above sample occurred in 2 min.
_____ **4.** Words per minute if the above sample occurred in 1 min.

Answers to Activities

17–1.

1. 54
2. 5
3. 2
4. 2
5. 1
6. 19% (10 total disfluencies divided by 54 total words = .1851 × 100 = 19%)
7. 22% (2 part-word repetitions divided by 10 total disfluencies = .20 × 100 = 20% part-word repetitions)

17–2.

1. 94 (47 × 2)
2. 141 (47 × 3)
3. 23.5 (47 / 2)
4. 47

Wrap-Up

1. Look at The Stuttering Foundation website (http://stutteringhelp.org). Go to the link for speech-language pathologists. Look at the links for determining eligibility in schools. In your own words, explain at least two criteria that must occur to consider a school-age child eligible for services. You may also find information regarding eligibility on the American Speech-Language-Hearing Association website and the Department of Public Instruction for the state in which you intend to practice.

_____
_____
_____
_____
_____

2. Look online at a video of childhood disfluency, a video of adult disfluency, and a video of cluttering. What disfluencies did you notice? How easy or difficult was it for you to pick out the disfluencies? What emotions did you experience while watching the videos? What similarities or differences did you notice? Transcribe parts of each video; what calculations can you make? What other things would you want to do if you were evaluating each of the people in the videos?

Disfluencies noted/ease of identification of disfluencies:

Video 1:

Video 2:

Video 3:

Emotions while you watched videos:

Similarities between videos:

Difference between videos:

Transcription of video 1:

Transcription of video 2:

Transcription of video 3:

Other evaluation methods would you like to use or questions you would ask.

References

Centers for Medicare and Medicaid Services (n.d.). Privacy and security information. Retrieved September 12, 2017, from https://www.cms.gov/Regulations-and-Guidance/Administrative-Simplification/HIPAA-ACA/PrivacyandSecurityInformation.html

Robinson, T. L., & Crowe, T. A. (1998). Culture-based considerations in programming for stuttering intervention with African American clients and their families. *Language, Speech and Hearing Services in Schools, 29*, 172–179.

Shipley, K. G., & McAfee, J. G. (2016). *Assessment in speech-language pathology* (5th ed.). Boston, MA: Cengage Learning.

U.S. Department of Health and Human Services. (n.d.). HIPAA for professionals. Retrieved April 20, 2018, from https://www.hhs.gov/hipaa/for-professionals/security/laws-regulations/index.html

Yaruss, J. S., & Quesal, R. W. (2008). *Overall assessment of the speaker's experience of stuttering*. Minneapolis, MN: NCS Pearson, Inc.

CHAPTER 18

Dysphagia Assessment

Who

The 2014 American Speech-Language-Hearing Association's (ASHA) standards for certification require competency and skills in diagnosing and treating dysphagia (American Speech-Language-Hearing Association, n.d.). There are also special certifications that can be obtained through the American Board of Swallowing and Swallowing Disorders (ASHA, 2014). While special certifications are not needed to asses and manage dysphagia as it is under the scope of practice of every speech-language pathologist (SLP), additional training is highly recommended. Speech-language pathologists are often asked to evaluate a person's swallowing ability, identify the presence and location of dysphagia, and rule out the risks or presence of aspiration (Golper, 2010).

Dysphagia can occur as a solitary problem or in conjunction with other communication or neurological disorders. Problems with swallowing can occur at any age. Dysphagia is a potentially life-threatening disorder, so extreme caution should be taken when evaluating and diagnosing patients with suspected dysphagia.

What

Clinicians should be familiar with and understand the terminology and phases of the normal swallowing process. The first phase, also known as the oral preparatory phase, is when the food (also referred to as bolus after being chewed) or liquid is going through the oral cavity. In this phase, a person is preparing their food or liquid for movement toward the stomach. The second phase, oral phase, is when the tongue moves the bolus or liquid toward the back of the mouth. The third phase, or pharyngeal phase, triggers the swallow reflex and moves the bolus or liquid through the laryngeal cavity. The final phase, esophageal phase, is when the bolus or liquid is traveling through the esophagus and into the stomach. This book is certainly not intended to give readers all the information they would need to perform a dysphagia exam, but rather to cover basic information that could be helpful in completing a dysphagia exam. The above information is only a synopsis of a normal swallow.

As with any other evaluation that may have been discussed in this workbook, a screening can be performed prior to a complete evaluation. A dysphagia screening can be done in a variety of ways so that the clinician can determine if a more thorough evaluation is recommended/needed. Again, due to the safety issues surrounding dysphagia, clinicians are encouraged to err on the side of caution and if there are any doubts that a patient has a normal swallow, they should be referred for more follow-up testing. During the time between a screening and a full evaluation, it is appropriate to make safety recommendations (i.e., nothing by mouth or specific dietary cautions) (ASHA, 2014).

When performing a dysphagia evaluation, the clinician will need to determine in which stage(s) the disorder is occurring. Determining this information can be done in a variety of ways including interview, questionnaires, observation, and administration of specific swallowing tasks. These steps will be discussed in detail in the How section. It is also important for the clinician to keep cultural competence in mind when performing a swallowing evaluation. If there are dietary restrictions or customs that are observed by a patient, those should be followed during the evaluation process.

Why

Clinicians must determine the swallowing abilities of a patient in order to ensure safety. Dysphagia is one of the areas of speech pathology in which a patient could end up in a critical situation if not diagnosed and treated correctly. While clinicians cannot force patients to adhere to recommendations, it is the responsibility of the clinician to properly assess and explain the results and recommendations to the patient.

When

Dysphagia screenings and/or evaluations should be completed anytime someone is concerned about or exhibiting problems with their ability to swallow. Some particular known instances of increased dysphagia problems involve the following populations: premature babies, patients with medical diagnoses or treatment of certain head/neck cancers, stroke patients, patients taking certain medications, as well as individuals with intellectual disorders, gastroesophageal reflux disease, and progressive neurological diseases.

Because eating is often a social situation and highly correlated to quality of life, it is important to remember that changing a patient's dietary habits can have additional complications or negative effects. A clinician will want to first ensure the safety of their patients, but also remember that treatment efforts should be made that allow a patient to quickly return to their regular eating habits or as close as safely possible.

Where

Swallowing evaluations can occur in a variety of settings including at a patient's bedside or in a clinic or hospital. Depending on the type of equipment needed, the evaluation may be done in a combination of settings.

How

There are many ways to complete a dysphagia examination. There are assessment techniques that do not rely on instrumentation and some that do. Noninstrumental techniques can be very effective in determining problems that are present in the first two stages of swallowing, but are generally less effective when the bolus/liquid reaches the level of the swallow reflex and beyond.

Case history and oral-facial examinations are helpful in determining if a client has strong indicators of swallowing problems or perceptions that they are struggling with swallowing. If a patient is in a medical setting, the clinician should also discuss concerns with the physician or nurse. Identifying the patient's current status of food or liquid intake is helpful in determining complications that have been noted, such as the patient fatiguing and then having difficulty with food or liquid intake. Oral-facial examination should follow the initial step of gathering information (see Chapter 4, Oral-Facial Examinations).

A bedside examination is done by presenting small bites or sips of various textures of food and/or liquids and making observations about the swallowing process. The bedside assessment should begin with easier to manage consistencies (i.e., pureed food, which has the same consistency throughout like mashed potatoes), then move to soft textured foods (ground or chopped foods), and finally, move to regular textured foods. Liquids may follow as they are more difficult to manage due to the lack of substance felt in the oral cavity and small amount of time to prepare the oral/pharyngeal cavity for the swallow; thus, a patient must rely on voluntary and reflexive movements to safely swallow. Liquids should be given to the patient only if it is safe to do so and should be given from a spoon, then a straw, then a cup. The clinician should observe any difficulties related to any of the four stages of the swallow. For example, food spilling from the lips indicates a problem with the oral preparatory phase, food pocketed in the buccal cavity is indicative of a problem in the oral phase, a wet sounding or gurgling voice is indicative of a problem in the pharyngeal stage, and coughing could be indicative of a problem in the esophageal stage. Again, it should be noted that these particular examples could occur in more than one stage, but with any of the examples, dysphagia should be suspected. There are specialized populations, including patients with tracheostomies, who would need modifications to the assessment process explained previously. While this workbook will not cover the specifics, it should be noted that clinicians should want to familiarize themselves with the Modified Evans Blue Dye Test (often referred to as the blue dye test) (Shipley & McAfee, 2016). Helpful checklists are available for use during a bedside evaluation. These checklists assist the clinician in systematically and efficiently conducting a bedside evaluation. Checklists will often cover information from case history, observation, and swallowing examination.

Instrumental tests include videoendoscopy and videofluroscopy. Videoendoscopy uses a technique called the fiberoptic endoscopic examination of swallow (FEES). In this procedure, a flexible endoscope is inserted in the nasal cavity and passes through to the level of the soft palate while the clinician provides various consistencies of food and liquid to the patient. This allows the clinician to view the pharyngeal and laryngeal structures before and after a swallow. The oral phases and esophageal phase are not visible using this method as there is no way to see the food being chewed and forming a bolus or liquid passing through the oral cavity, nor can the clinician see the bolus traveling through the esophageal stage. This method is helpful for determining areas of concern just prior to and after the swallow occurs. FEES is typically portable so it can be transported the patient's bedside and does not have any need for radiography involvement. A clinician should be adequately trained in the use of the equipment and should have achieved a level of competence prior to using this method. Some states have specific certification requirements; therefore, clinicians should check with their particular state licensing boards to determine guidelines surrounding use of this equipment.

Videofluoroscopy is also known as a videofluorographic swallow study (VFSS) or modified barium swallow study (MBSS). This evaluation tool is a radiographic procedure that provides a direct, dynamic view of oral, pharyngeal, and upper esophageal function (Logemann, 1998). The clinician would provide the patient with various consistencies of food and liquid that are mixed with barium, which allows for the visualization of the entire swallowing process using live x-ray techniques. This method allows a clinician to more accurately assess the occurrence of silent aspiration. Silent aspiration occurs when food and or liquid pass through to the lungs without outward indications such as coughing. This can occur when a patient's anatomical structures or the neural message is not working properly to protect the airway during swallowing. Silent aspiration can lead to aspiration pneumonia as food and or liquid enters the lungs. When performing VFSS/MBSS, an SLP and radiologist will work together. While the code of ethics provided by ASHA for SLPs addresses these tests being completed without a radiologist, best practice would be to have both professions present during the study. There are again specific state guidelines clinicians should be familiar with before beginning these tests. Following the review of the tests, a clinician will need to determine at what level dysphagia is occurring, which is often called scaling the swallow. It should be noted that from clinician to clinician there may be differences in the terminology used to scale the swallow. Because of variation, one tool that has been developed is the penetration-aspiration (PA) scale (Coyle, 2017). This tool can be used to bring more standardization across clinic settings and may be a beneficial tool for clinicians to explore.

Top 10 Terms

Dysphagia

Oral preparatory stage

Oral stage

Pharyngeal stage

Esophageal stage

Bedside examination

Pureed food

FEES

VFSS/MBSS

Silent aspiration

Chapter Tips

1. Dysphagia can occur at any age. Extreme caution should be taken when determining dysphagia as this could be a life-threatening disorder.
2. Observation plays a large role in the dysphagia evaluation.
3. Instrumental assessments fall under the scope of practice for an SLP; however, there may be specific state guidelines regarding using these procedures.

Activities

18–1. Determine the stage(s) of swallowing based on the following descriptions of difficulties:

_____ 1. Coughing

_____ 2. Excessive chewing time

_____ 3. Regurgitation of bolus due to cricopharyngeal dysfunction

_____ 4. Nasal regurgitation due to poor velopharyngeal closure

_____ 5. Spillage of food due to poor labial seal

_____ 6. Residual food is left on the hard palate after swallow due to poor lingual elevation

18–2. Using the following case history, determine what questions you would want answered prior to beginning a swallowing evaluation.

Tulifinny, an 80-year-old-female in a skilled nursing facility, has recently started experiencing "coughing fits" while drinking her morning coffee at breakfast. The nurses have noticed she has been very lethargic in the morning, often taking her until almost lunchtime before she starts acting like her normal self.

Potential questions:

#1:

_____
_____
_____

#2:

#3:

Answers to Activities

18–1.

1. Pharyngeal and/or esophageal stage
2. Oral preparatory stage
3. Esophageal stage
4. Pharyngeal stage
5. Oral preparatory stage
6. Oral stage

18–2.

1. Are there any other times of the day when she is experiencing these "coughing fits"? Does it only occur when she is drinking her coffee? When she eats food?
2. Have there been any noted medical or pharmacological changes in the last few weeks/months?
3. Is she experiencing any other medical conditions? Is she concerned about swallowing and/or drinking her coffee in the mornings now?

Wrap-Up

1. Watch two videos of FEES testing. Now watch two videos of VFSS/MBSS testing. What pros/cons can you determine about each test? Think of contraindications to these types of tests. Can you think of other testing methods that could be used? Would these other methods yield the same information?

Pros of FEES:

Cons of FEES:

Pros of VFSS/MBSS:

Cons of VFSS/MBSS:

Contraindications to FEES:

Contraindications to VFSS/MBSS:

Other possible tests and would they yield the same information:

2. Look online at four examples of a bedside swallowing evaluation. What is your favorite and why? Using information from those examples, develop a bedside evaluation checklist. Do not forget to include patient information/questions at the top.

Bedside Evaluation Checklist

Demographic information:

Oral-facial examination/observations:

Pharyngeal/laryngeal examination/observations:

_____

_____

_____

_____

_____

_____

_____

_____

_____

Swallow evaluation:

_____

_____

_____

_____

_____

_____

_____

_____

_____

3. Take the information on dysphagia assessment a step further. What could/should you do if a patient is deemed to have an unsafe swallow, yet they do not adhere to your recommendations? What are your ethical obligations? Think through how you could provide additional information to the patient to help them understand the gravity of continuing to eat/drink foods/liquids that are not recommended?

_____

_____

_____

_____

References

American Speech-Language-Hearing Association (n.d.) Adult dysphagia assessment. Retrieved December 21, 2017, from http://www.asha.org/PRPSpecificTopic.aspx?folderid=8589942550&section=Assessment

Coyle, J. L. (2017). Scaling the swallow. *The ASHA Leader, 22*(5), 36–38.

Golper, L. A. (2010). *Medical speech-language pathology: A desk reference* (3rd ed.). Clifton Park, NY: Delmar.

Loggemann, J. A. (1998). *Evaluation and treatment of swallowing disorders* (2nd ed.). Austin, TX.: Pro-Ed, Inc.

Shipley, K. G., & McAfee, J. G. (2016) *Assessment in speech-language pathology* (5th ed.). Boston, MA: Cengage Learning.

CHAPTER 19

Language/Literacy in Children

Who

Language/literacy assessment is highly connected to the age of the client being assessed. Children born with a physical disability, sensory disability, multiple disabilities, or a syndrome are often identified as infants. Since a language/literacy component is common with these diagnoses, language will be evaluated early as part of the total evaluation. In the past, children suspected of having autism were often not evaluated until preschool age (3–5 years old). Today, identification of key social milestones for children between 9 and 16 months old has been recognized to aid in early identification of autism spectrum disorders (Wetherby, 2017). As a profession, we recognize that the earlier we can identify and treat a language or literacy disorder, the better our outcome.

Preschool age remains a time when language/literacy problems are most commonly detected by family members, teachers, and physicians and referrals for evaluations are made. At this young age, a noncategorical diagnosis can be made, essentially identifying a speech/language disorder without labeling a disability category.

Assessment in the schools takes an academic focus, as a language/literacy disorder may have a negative impact on educational learning. Evaluation of culturally and linguistically diverse students to determine if they demonstrate a difference or a disorder in their speech and language is also a role clinicians serve in the schools.

Team assessment is common when a child has suspected language/literacy issues. The assessment may be done in an interdisciplinary manner, with each professional assessing separately at different times using different procedures and sharing their findings in a transdisciplinary manner. This would involve multiple individuals representing several disciplines evaluating the same interaction and building their findings together.

Regardless of the child's age or format of the assessment, the speech/language clinician serves as a model of language production. It is important that a clinician uses appropriate grammar (syntax), vocabulary (semantics), nonverbal communication (pragmatics), and sound system (phonology). We urge all students in training to seek treatment for any speech/language disorders they may have. Training programs typically provide assistance in these areas. Do not be embarrassed or hesitate to seek help. Your ability to serve as a speech/language model is important. In addition, experiencing assessment and treatment from the client's perspective can give you new insight.

What

Typically, language is evaluated by splitting it into the components of syntax and morphology, semantics, pragmatics, and phonology. Standardized tests are often structured to assess these language areas separately through receptive and/or expressive tasks (e.g., Preschool Language Scales, Fifth Edition, by Zimmerman, Steiner, & Pond, 2011). The standardized testing is then followed by an authentic assessment such as a language sample, a conversational observation, and/or a structured interaction with the clinician to integrate all the components of language. Likewise, literacy evaluations segment the skills needed for reading and writing in the standardized testing process (e.g., Assessment of Literacy and Language, Lombardino, Lieberman, & Brown, 2009) and then recombine the segmented factors.

Standardized language/literacy tests vary in their purpose. Some are screening tests used to help determine if additional testing is needed (e.g., Bankson Language Screening Test, Bankson, 1990). Some are broad-based tests examining an array of areas and focusing on both receptive and expressive skills (e.g., Clinical Evaluation of Language Fundamentals, Fifth Edition, Wiig, Semel, & Secord, 2013). Some tests are specifically focused on a single area, such as receptive vocabulary use (e.g., Peabody Picture Vocabulary Test, Fourth Edition, Dunn & Dunn, 2007) or word finding examination (e.g., Test of Word Finding, Third Edition, German, 2015), to provide more comprehensive information on a specific area of concern. The clinician should select the test(s) best suited to answer the diagnostic question(s) driving the assessment. Language/literacy assessments should always include an actual communication interaction examination and not be limited to fragmented skill tasks.

The authentic component of the evaluation can take on a variety of forms. A representative sample of oral and/or written language can provide valuable information to any language/literacy evaluation. Samples taken in both the primary and secondary languages are especially valuable when assessing culturally and linguistically diverse children, and knowing the characteristics of both languages is necessary for analyzing the language samples of this population. Observations and structured interactions with the clinician can also be used to provide the integrated look at language skills needed for a comprehensive evaluation.

Dynamic assessment—including trials of therapy techniques, data collection on multiple relevant items, and discussion of reasoning with clients—provides the details needed for establishing recommended goals and objectives. Dynamic assessment also provides valuable insight needed for the differential diagnosis with culturally and linguistically diverse children. Together, these formal and informal procedures of standardized testing, authentic assessment, and dynamic assessment tasks compose the basis for language/literacy assessment.

Why

Why we do language/literacy evaluation should be obvious. One's language and literacy skills permeate everything one does. Even when language is not central to the questions driving the assessment, it is still routinely screened.

When

Language screening is conducted whenever a clinician performs any speech/language/hearing/swallowing evaluation. This could involve a standardized screening test, a clinician-developed set of questions or probes, or observation of language use throughout the evaluation process. At the conclusion of a screening, a decision is made as to whether further assessment in the language area is needed.

Language is assessed when a referral for testing is received. Once an individual is enrolled in treatment, language skills continue to be monitored as appropriate and retesting is completed periodically.

Where

Language assessment is often done in various settings. Standardized testing is most commonly done on a one-to-one, clinician-to-client basis in a controlled environment (i.e., treatment or assessment room). At times, a language/literacy test may be designed to assess a group of individuals at the same time in a classroom setting such as the Boehm-3 (Boehm Test of Basic Concepts, Third Edition, Boehm, 2001). Multiple observations can and should be done across settings (e.g., science class, circle time, lunch and/or recess) and partners (e.g., peers, teachers, and/or family members). A language sample or samples can be set up in a therapy room or other settings. The communication partner can be the clinician, family member, peer, or teacher. A quality audio or video recording is desirable in a language sample; thus, many are taken in the controlled environment of the therapy room. A structured interview and dynamic assessment tasks, while possible in a classroom or home environment, are most commonly staged in a therapy room.

How

Preparation is key when completing a language/literacy evaluation. The following figures provide a series of checklists to help you prepare for giving the standardized test, authentic language sample or structured interaction, and the dynamic assessment.

Figure 19–1 provides a checklist a clinician could use when reviewing the standardized test manual prior to giving the language/literacy test.

Preparing to Use a Standardized Test Checklist

Put a check before each item to signify you know this information. Your test manual will be your guide to these questions.

Test name:_____

___ Can I articulate the stated purpose of the test?

___ Am I qualified to give this test according to the manual?

___ Do I have all the facts to complete the client information on the test score form?

___ Is my client within the ages for which the test is normed?

___ On what number item do I start for this client?

___ If there is a specified basal, what do I do if he/she does not meet the qualifications required in the basal?

___ On what number item do I end (e.g., 8 errors in a row or the last question on the test)?

___ Do I know the difference in my behavior when giving trial items versus scored items?

___ Can I repeat an item if the client does not respond or asks for a repetition?

___ Do I understand the score sheet–where and what do I mark on the form as I give the test?

___ Do I understand the summary information I record on the test form? Do I know where the needed tables in the test manual are located?

___ Do I plan to give the test in its entirety?

Figure 19–1. Clinician checklist for reviewing the test manual.

Preparing to Use an Authentic Measure Checklist

Put a check before each item to signify you know this information.

Description of authentic measure planned: _____

___ Can I articulate the stated purpose of authentic measure?

___ If taking a language sample:

   ___ Do I have age appropriate materials that support more than just naming responses?

   ___ Do I have permission to audio or video tape the child?

   ___ Do I have an audio or video recorder so I can transcribe all speakers and context of the interaction?

   ___ Do I know how many utterances I wish to analyze?

   ___ Can I explain to conversational partner their role?

   ___ If I am to be the partner, am I prepared to make comments or ask open ended questions to elicit a representative sample?

   ___ Do I know how to transcribe a sample in an organized manner (e.g. the left column for the partner's output, the middle column for context notes, and the right column for the clients output)?

   ___ Do I know how to determine such measures as mean length of utterance (MLU), type toke ration (TTR), semantic categories, and pragmatic skills (e.g., topic initiation, topic maintenance, eye contact etc.)?

___ If I am conducting an observation:

   ___ Do I have age appropriate materials available for the interaction?

   ___ Do I have permission to audio or video tape the child and partner?

   ___ Have I selected the setting and arranged to observe in that setting?

Figure 19–2. Clinician checklist for planning the authentic component of an assessment.

___ Do I have an audio or video recorder or am I prepared to do verbatim live transcription or take organized notes?
___ Do I know what I am focusing on in the observation?
___ Do I have a time frame for this observation?
___ If I am conducting a structured interaction:
  ___ Do I have age appropriate materials available for the interaction?
  ___ Do I have permission to audio or video tape the child?
  ___ Do I have a focus for the structured interaction (e.g., if intentional communication with a young child is the focus have I considered the Communication Temptations by Wetherby and Prizant (1989)?
  ___ Have I planned how I will set-up, deliver, and analyze the structured interactions?
  ___ Have I developed a recording sheet to help me stay focused and organized during the interaction?
  ___ Do I have a time frame for the structured interaction?

Figure 19–2. (*continued*)

Preparing to Use a Dynamic Measure Checklist

Put a check before each item to signify you know this information. Concept to be assessed: _____

___ Do I have age appropriate materials available for the dynamic task?
___ Have I determined steps I will use to assess including a discussion with the client as to the reasons for his response?
___ Do I know how I will analyze the results (change in test-teach-test format or perhaps a cueing hierarchy rating or a measure of examiner effort)?
___ Have I considered recommendations for interpreting the results (if this happens then this is the recommendation)?
___ Have I planned to collect sufficient data to set my goals and objective?
___ Have I developed a recording sheet to help me stay focused and organized during the dynamic assessment?
___ Do I have a time frame for the dynamic interaction?

Figure 19–3. Clinician checklist for planning the dynamic component of an assessment.

Figure 19–2 provides a checklist a clinician could use when planning the authentic component of the language assessment.

Figure 19–3 provides a checklist a clinician could use when planning the dynamic component of the language assessment.

Top 10 Terms

Authentic assessment

Communication temptations

Dynamic assessment

Interdisciplinary

Language

Language sample analyses (i.e., MLU, TTR, pragmatic skills)

Literacy

Noncategorical

Preliteracy skills

Transdisciplinary

Chapter Tips

1. An error some beginning clinicians make is giving a narrowly focused test and over applying the results to make a conclusion about overall language skills. Be careful. If you test only receptive skills, you cannot use them to draw conclusions about expressive skills. In a descriptive look at a clinical case of ineffective language remediation, Damico (1988) identified fragmenting of language when assessing as an important contributing factor. Assessment needs to go beyond static tests to provide a valid view of the client's abilities.

2. Use your team to provide a more complete picture of a child's language/literacy skills than you have acquired from your limited assessment time.

3. Dyslexia is frequently associated with a history of ear infections, phonological errors, and delayed syntactic skills (Research in Brief, 2018). Make sure your assessment includes hearing, language, phonology, fluency, and voice screenings.

Activities

19–1. A clinician needs to be a good language model by using appropriate grammar, vocabulary, pragmatics, and speech sound production. In the following sentences, write CORRECT if the grammar is standard English; but if there are any grammatical errors, rewrite the sentence correcting those errors.

1. Me and my supervisor appreciate you coming in today.
2. We have acquired some additional funding at the clinic and are able to provide services at a reduced rate.
3. I had did the observation of your child last week in his classroom.
4. I and the whole early childhood team have examined the results of Andy's assessment.
5. I will get that report wrote up for you and send it within 7 days.

19–2. Match the description of the concern given by the referral source to the specific language area you would emphasize in the assessment. The areas to select from are receptive semantics, expressive semantics, expressive syntax, receptive syntax, expressive pragmatics, and receptive pragmatics.

1. _____ Carmen's speech is clear and her grammar is usually correct. She seems to jump around in her conversation. One day she was talking about her sister and said, "She had three kittens." She had switched to talking about her cat.

2. _____ Henry has difficulty following direction in written or oral form. He confuses the meaning of opposite words like top and bottom or right and left.

3. _____ Franklin leaves off the *s* sound in plurals and possessive words, although he can say the *s* in "boss."

4. _____ Bert understands things said to him, but when he talks, he uses nonspecific words like, "like," "kind of," "that thing," and "you know."

19–3. Name two appropriate materials you would use for taking a language sample or doing a conversational observation at each age listed and two you would not choose to use. Then, provide the reason you would not use the second set of materials.

Age 2 to 3: I would use _____ and _____.
I would not use _____ and _____ because _____.

Age 5 to 6: I would use _____ and _____.
I would not use _____ and _____ because _____.

Age 10 to 12: I would use _____ and _____.
I would not use _____ and _____ because _____.

Age 15 to 16: I would use _____ and _____.
I would not use _____ and _____ because _____.

Answers to Activities

19–1

1. My supervisor and I appreciate you coming in today.
2. CORRECT
3. I did the observation of your child last week in his classroom.
4. The whole early childhood team and I have examined the results of Andy's assessment.
5. I will get that report written up for you and send it within 7 days.

19–2.

1. Expressive pragmatics
2. Receptive semantics
3. Expressive syntax
4. Expressive semantics

19–3.

Note. Answers may vary; these are some suggestions. We selected a reading item in each case.

Age 2 to 3: I would use **bubbles** and **an age-appropriate book**.

I would not use **cars** and **musical items** because **cars tend to lead to noise sounds, not words,** and **musical items do not promote talking**.

Age 5 to 6: I would use **birthday party things** and **an age-appropriate book; maybe one with a story but no words like *Frog Goes to Dinner* by Mercer Mayer**.

I would not use **blocks** and **flash cards** because **blocks and flash cards do not promote conversation**.

Age 10 to 12: I would use **a game for the client to give me directions on how to play** and **an age-appropriate book**.

I would not use **video games** and **school texts** because **video games do not promote interacting** and **school texts are not the most engaging**.

Age 15 to 16: I would use **topic cards for the client to select from** and **a driving manual**.

I would not use **a physical game** and **school texts** because **physical games do not tend to promote conversation** and **school texts are not the most engaging**.

Wrap-Up

1. Set the timer on your phone for 2 min. Write down the names of all the language/literacy tests you can. Use the examples from the chapter, the internet, or textbooks to add three additional tests to your list.

   _____
   _____
   _____
   _____

2. Should a clinician be encouraged to use his/her dialect in assessment sessions if it varies from standard English? Identify the pros and cons of this issue.

   Pros:
   _____
   _____

   Cons:
   _____
   _____

3. "Eat a desired food item in front of your child without offering any to him/her" is one of the communication temptations from Wetherby and Prizant (1989). Name an appropriate verbal response, an appropriate nonverbal response, an inappropriate verbal response, and an inappropriate nonverbal response from a 2-year-old child.

   Appropriate verbal response:
   _____

   Appropriate nonverbal response:
   _____

   Inappropriate verbal response:
   _____

   Inappropriate nonverbal response:
   _____

4. If you were going to print a T-shirt with a motto from the language/literacy assessment chapter what would it say?
   _____
   _____

References

Bankson, N. W. (1990). Bankson language screening test [Assessment instrument]. Austin, TX: Pro-Ed.

Boehm, A. E. (2001). Boehm test of basic concepts (3rd ed.) [Assessment instrument]. San Antonio, TX: Pearson.

Damico, J. S. (1988). The lack of efficacy in language therapy: A case study. *Language Speech, Hearing in Schools, 19*, 51–66.

Dunn, L. M., & Dunn, D. M, (2007). Peabody picture vocabulary test (4th ed.) [Assessment instrument]. San Antonio, TX: Pearson.

German, D. (2015). Test of word finding (3rd ed.) [Assessment instrument]. Austin, TX: Pro-Ed.

Lombardino, L. J., Lieberman, R. J., & Brown, J. J. (2009). Assessment of literacy and language [Assessment instrument]. San Antonio, TX: Pearson.

Mayer, M. (1974) *Frog goes to dinner*. New York, NY: Dial Press.

Research in Brief. (2018). Children with dyslexia or repeated ear infections may struggle with phonology. *The ASHA Leader, 23*, 14.

Wetherby, A. M. (2017, March). *Mobilizing community systems to improve early detection & change developmental trajectories of toddlers with autism spectrum disorders: Strategies for bridging research to practice*. Presented at the Cullowhee Conference on Communicative Disorders, Cullowhee, NC. Retrieved from https://www.wcu.edu/WebFiles/PDFs/WetherbyWCUSlidestoPost32417.pdf

Wetherby A. M., & Prizant, B. (1989). EC handout #8 Valley CoPA (Community of Practice in Autism). Retrieved from http://www.infantva.org/documents/CoPA-Jan-8-CommTempt%20WPrizant.pdf

Wiig, E. H., Semel, E., & Secord, W. A. (2013). Clinical evaluation of language fundamentals (5th ed.) [Assessment instrument]. San Antonio, TX: Pearson.

Zimmerman, I. L., Steiner, V. G., & Pond, R. E. (2011). Preschool language scales (5th ed.) [Assessment instrument]. San Antonio, TX: Pearson.

CHAPTER 20

Adult Language Assessment

Who

Neurological issues can cause difficulties with communication for adults. This chapter will focus on aphasia and right hemisphere syndrome and their relationship to language disorders for adults. There are other diagnoses for adults such as apraxia and dysarthria; however, these are motor speech disorders as opposed to language disorders. There are also issues such as traumatic brain injury and dementia; however, these issues will be discussed in the cognitive assessment chapter (Chapter 21).

What

Aphasia is a language disorder that occurs due to some type of brain damage. Most often, this occurs because of a stroke but can be caused by traumatic brain injury, brain tumors, or other neurological conditions. Aphasia can be evident with problems with receptive language, expressive language, or a combination of language problems. It can be difficult for someone with aphasia to understand language and/or use speech/language to communicate. Typically, aphasia occurs as a result of damage to the left side of the brain, as this is where the language centers are located; however, right hemisphere damage can also lead to language issues such as word retrieval problems, reading and writing issues, and difficulty with pragmatics.

Every patient will be different as determined by the site of lesion, the severity of the injury, as well as additional factors such as time between onset and treatment for the injury. Spontaneous recovery can occur and will also be different from patient to patient. Spontaneous recovery is the recovery that occurs without treatment. Because patients vary so much, it is difficult to determine a set of specific behaviors or deficits to look for. While there is no one way to properly identify aphasia and no one agreed upon way to classify aphasia, there are some overarching areas that make it easier to categorize a person and their communicative problems.

Categorizing aphasia into nonfluent aphasia and fluent aphasia is a widely accepted practice. The American Speech-Language-Hearing Association (ASHA) describes nonfluent aphasia as speech production being effortful with grammar impairments and likelihood of intact content words (Aphasia, n.d.). Fluent aphasia has been described as sentence structure being relatively intact but lacking meaning (Shipley & McAfee, 2016). Other characteristics that are commonly tied to aphasia are anomia (problems finding and naming words), impaired reading and writing ability, impaired auditory comprehension, and impaired verbal expression. A recent study by Salis, Murray, and Bakas (2018) indicated it is also important to determine the short-term memory and working memory of a patient with aphasia in order to get a broader picture of their abilities. Once again, it is important to remember that every patient will be different and a holistic assessment should be completed to determine strengths and weaknesses with anyone suspected of having aphasia or right hemisphere disorders.

Why

Because every patient exhibiting adult language disorders has the potential to have different problems and severities, a comprehensive assessment is vital for the proper diagnosis and treatment.

Most often, patients who are exhibiting language impairments as an adult will have had typical language skills and experienced an event that has caused problems with their ability to communicate. This can happen fast and be devastating to the patient and family members/friends. Acting quickly to assess language problems and determining proper treatment can make a difference in the length and amount of recovery a patient can expect.

When

The assessment process should begin as soon as concerns have been identified. Acting quickly can be vital in the recovery of language abilities when a person has experienced a stroke. Concerning other neurological issues, assessment should still occur as quickly as possible in order to assist a patient with determining appropriate goals and strategies to implement.

Sometimes in cases of other medical issues, the speech/language evaluation process may have to wait as other more pressing medical situations must be dealt with. If a person is having difficulty swallowing, a dysphagia examination may take precedence over the language evaluation. Not that multiple evaluations cannot be done during the same time frame, but the medical team must prioritize issues and providers should adhere to those decisions.

Where

Adult language evaluations can take place in a variety of settings. Most often clinicians will conduct screenings to determine the need for a full evaluation. Screenings often take place in the hospital or rehabilitation facility after a person has been discharged from the hospital. In some instances, the assessment may have to wait until other issues have been taken care of, and therefore the assessment will be completed at a skilled nursing facility, the home, or a clinic setting.

How

As always, case history and interviews will be important tools in the assessment process. When working with adults, clinicians have the ability to gather information from the client, family members, and/or others who are familiar with the patient. When working with adult language disorders, it is important to keep in mind that with some types of aphasia it could be very difficult for the patient to respond; but, most often, the cognitive abilities are not affected.

When dealing with adults there are several things to keep in mind prior to testing. Hearing loss is more prevalent in this population and even if a patient does not report hearing loss, it does not mean they do not have hearing loss. If a patient wears hearing aids, you want to make sure they are wearing them during the evaluation if possible. Not hearing the question correctly can cause a patient to answer incorrectly; thus, making it look like they have deficits with language when perhaps they do not. You want to make sure you are testing in an environment that is as quiet and well-lit as possible. Vision loss is also prevalent in the adult population. When testing, you want to make sure the patient is wearing their appropriate glasses as well as other medical or dental devices, in order to make sure you are assessing the client's true language abilities. Again, as a clinician, you want to obtain valid and reliable results so some planning and preparation prior to the assessment is important.

Case history and self-reporting can give you information on the patient's medical status, occupation, education, current medications, cultural/linguistic background, as well as his/her areas of concern and goals he/she hopes to achieve. Sometimes you may be gathering this information through medical documents or self-report forms. You may also need to ask follow-up questions or take the opportunity to do a patient/family interview as part of the assessment.

Oral-motor examinations are another important component of the assessment. While this chapter focuses on the language aspects for adults, it is important for the clinician to gather this vital information on oral strength, speed, and range of motion. Language disorders in adults can occur alone or with other disorders such as apraxia or swallowing difficulties.

There are many standardized language tests available on the market for assessing adult language disorders. Typically, when assessing adult language, you want to obtain information on the patient's expressive language and receptive language skills for both spoken and written language. Testing items often consist of things such as memory, auditory comprehension, yes–no questions, sentence and reading comprehension, repetition, writing, and naming. Some tests use a classification model, meaning that upon obtaining the results, the clinician will be able to use the score to determine a certain type or level of deficit. Other tests do not consist of a classification system but rather rank the patient on abilities and problem areas. There are other standardized tests that make a prognostic statement using the test results. This means that based on the patient's scores, the clinician can determine a typical prognosis for the patient.

When looking at pragmatics, a language analysis or observation could be used. Most language tests do not include a thorough pragmatic piece, so this additional information is helpful in determining skills and treatment direction.

Often when testing adults, the clinician may be using pictures or items. Typically, in this scenario, the clinician would give the patient a picture or object, ask them to name it, and have the patient explain its use. A task such as this would allow the clinician to assess a few different areas in a short amount of time. In order to complete tasks such as this, the clinician will need to make sure they have the appropriate pictures or items and consider using preprinted checklists to make the process move more quickly and systematically. Currently, there is no standardized test of word retrieval in discourse for persons with aphasia, which makes it challenging to measure change in performance (Boyle, 2014).

As with other disorder areas that have been discussed in this workbook, screenings can be completed initially to determine if a full evaluation is warranted. Screenings are often done in an acute setting at the bedside or as soon as a patient is in a rehabilitation facility. Because screenings are not comprehensive but rather allow a clinician to determine if a full evaluation is warranted, the clinician should have a protocol in place that includes observational data as well as standardized assessment data.

Top 10 Terms

Aphasia

Right hemisphere syndrome (involvement)

Site of lesion

Nonfluent aphasia

Fluent aphasia

Classification system

Prognostic statements

Neurological syndrome

Stroke

Traumatic brain injury

Chapter Tips

1. Aphasia is the result of a brain injury. The injury is most often in the left hemisphere as this is where the language centers of the brain are located; however, right hemisphere problems can lead to language deficits as well.

2. Assessments should evaluate the patient's strengths and weaknesses in both expressive and receptive language areas for spoken and written language.

3. Knowing the status of the patient's hearing and vision will help make sure a patient is not given a misdiagnosis because they cannot hear or understand the test items or directions.

Activities

20–1. Read the following tasks and determine if they are testing expressive language speaking, receptive language nonverbal, receptive language reading, receptive language speaking, or expressive language writing (more than one area may be assessed with a task).

_____ 1. "Point to the flower" (when shown a page of pictures).

_____ 2. "Name these items" (when given a page of pictures and clinician is pointing to various pictures).

_____ 3. "Touch your nose."

_____ 4. "Put the spoon on the box."

_____ 5. Give the patient a short sentence and have them read it.

_____ 6. Ask yes or no questions about a short paragraph you have read aloud.

_____ 7. Give the patient a picture and have them tell you what is happening.

_____ 8. Ask the patient to write the words you say.

_____ 9. Ask the patient to point to items in the room.

_____ 10. Ask the patient to match written words to pictures.

20–2. Order the following list to show the order of the steps to prepare for and complete an adult language assessment (this is not all inclusive of all steps that should be taken).

_____ Choose a standardized assessment tool.

_____ Read medical chart.

_____ Review medication list.

_____ Talk with the patient about their case history.

_____ Develop a treatment plan.

_____ Review audiogram information.

_____ Determine an appropriate place to assess the patient.

_____ Score the assessment data.

_____ Analyze the language sample.

_____ Choose topics of conversation for the language sample.

_____ Complete an oral-motor examination.

Answers to Activities

20–1.

1. Receptive language nonverbal
2. Expressive language speaking
3. Receptive language nonverbal
4. Receptive language nonverbal
5. Receptive language reading
6. Receptive language speaking
7. Expressive language writing/receptive language nonverbal
8. Expressive language writing/receptive language nonverbal
9. Receptive language nonverbal
10. Receptive language reading/receptive language nonverbal

20–2.

6	Choose a standardized assessment tool.
1	Read medical chart.
2	Review medication list.
7	Talk with the patient about their case history.
11	Develop a treatment plan.
3	Review audiogram information.
4	Determine an appropriate place to assess the patient.
9	Score the assessment data.
10	Analyze the language sample.
5	Choose topics of conversation for the language sample.
8	Complete an oral-motor examination.

Wrap-Up

1. Watch video examples of the following types of aphasia: Wernicke's aphasia, Broca's aphasia, fluent aphasia, nonfluent aphasia, and right hemisphere stroke. Document the following:

   Describe the patient's language skills with Wernicke's aphasia:

   _____
   _____
   _____

Describe the patient's language skills with Broca's aphasia:

Describe the patient's language skills with fluent aphasia:

Describe the patient's language skills with nonfluent aphasia:

Describe the patient's language skills with right hemisphere stroke:

Similarities between videos/types of aphasia:

Differences between videos/types of aphasia:

_____

_____

_____

_____

_____

_____

_____

What evaluation methods would you like to use or questions would you ask?

_____

_____

_____

_____

_____

_____

_____

_____

References

Aphasia. (n.d.). Retrieved January 21, 2018, from https://www.asha.org/Practice-Portal/Clinical-Topics/Aphasia/

Boyle, M. (2014). Test-retest stability of word retrieval in aphasic discourse. *Journal of Speech, Language and Hearing Research, 57*(3), 966–978.

Salis, C., Murray, L., & Bakas, K. (2018). An international survey of assessment practices for short-term and working memory deficits in aphasia. *American Journal of Speech-Language Pathology, 27*(2), 574–591.

Shipley, K. G., & McAfee, J. G. (2016). *Assessment in speech-language pathology* (5th ed.). Boston, MA: Cengage Learning.

CHAPTER 21

Cognitive Assessment

Who

Cognitive assessments may need to be conducted for a variety of patients. Patients with intellectual disabilities may have concomitant speech and/or language deficits. Intellectual disabilities occur from birth to geriatrics and are primarily diagnosed prior to the age of 18 (unless an event causes some type of intellectual disorder). Other populations this chapter focuses on include patients with traumatic brain injury, which can occur at any age, and dementia patients. With any of the aforementioned disorders, the severity level can be mild to severe. With traumatic brain injury, the speech-language pathologist (SLP) may provide services that range from determining procedures explicitly aimed at improving orientation, attention, vigilance, and other cognitive functions to providing education and counseling to the patient and family members about the disorder and expected steps/course to recovery (Golper, 2010). As one can see, a clinician may be needed to provide information across a variety of areas when dealing with cognitive assessments and disorders.

What

Intellectual disabilities (ID) are defined by the American Speech-Language-Hearing Association (ASHA) as significant limitations in intellectual functioning and adaptive behavior that must be occur before age 18 (Intellectual Disabilities, n.d.). Limitations in intellectual functioning include things such as reasoning, problem-solving, and learning. Limitations in adaptive behavior include things like problems conceptualizing or adapting to situations in everyday life. A clinician may also see the term developmental disability (DD). This term, DD, is an overarching term that includes not only intellectual disabilities, but also could include other physical or emotional disabilities that result in substantial functional limitations in life activity.

Traumatic brain injury (TBI) is the result of an acute assault to the brain (Shipley & McAfee, 2016). There are two types of TBI, penetrating and closed-head injury. A penetrating injury occurs when an object penetrates the brain, while a closed-head injury occurs when the head collides with an object or surface that does not penetrate the brain. Penetrating injuries are localized to the area of the brain that has experienced the penetration (or point of impact). Closed-head injuries are not localized to one area as the brain collided against something and may have caused damage to more than just the area that was involved initially. TBI patients may experience a period of time when they are unconscious when the injury occurs. There are two rating scales that are often used when working with patients who have experienced a TBI. The Glasgow Coma Scale (GCS) assesses the level of consciousness following TBI (Shipley & McAfee, 2016). This scale evaluates eye opening, verbal response, and motor response. The patient is rated on a scale from 3 to 15, with lower scores being more severe. The Rancho Los Amigos Levels of Cognitive Functioning, also known as Rancho Levels, is designed to rate cognitive status using eight levels, with the lower levels indicating a more severe rating.

Dementia is an acquired brain disease and typically involves progressive deterioration in memory and other cognitive areas (Dementia, n.d.). Some neurodegenerative diseases that are associated with dementia include Alzheimer's disease, Huntington's disease, Parkinson's disease, and multiple sclerosis; additionally, some chemotherapy is associated with dementia. Generally, dementia progresses from mild to severe over the course of time. Dementia is often categorized into early dementia, intermediate dementia, and advanced dementia, with symptoms progressing and the ability to take care of oneself decreasing in each stage.

Why

Cognitive assessments are important to determine the current level of functioning for the patient. There are some cognitive issues in which spontaneous recovery could occur and other cognitive issues in which the disorder is progressive. A clinician must determine the strengths and weaknesses of a patient in order to recommend appropriate treatment.

When

Cognitive assessments may be done at any age. Early intervention is shown to be very beneficial; therefore, when cognitive problems are suspected in babies/children, a cognitive assessment should be completed. For school-age children (3–21 years old), cognitive assessments must be completed every three years to coincide with Individual Education Program (IEP) reevaluation dates. The three-year time is a maximum and children may have assessments completed prior to the three-year deadline. For adults or children with TBI, cognitive assessments are completed following an event or diagnosis that has identified a change in cognitive status. Cognitive assessments for adults may also be done if a patient is changing service providers or environments or has newly developed or identified strengths or weaknesses.

Where

Assessments may be completed in a variety of settings. Depending on the population, you may be completing an assessment in a clinic setting, classroom environment, home setting, hospital, skilled nursing facility, community setting, or group home.

How

As always, a complete assessment may begin as a screening that has indicated the need for a complete evaluation. Case history will be important information, along with interviews with family members and/or caregivers, other service providers, and the patient. Reviewing documentation such as results from hearing, visual, motor, and cognitive status is important as well (Traumatic Brain Injury, n.d.).

Assessments may be done using multidisciplinary, interdisciplinary, transdisciplinary, or interprofessional collaborative practice teams. Multidisciplinary teams share information but work separately and independently from one another. Interdisciplinary teams collaborate and communicate but focus on their own profession and testing from that perspective. Transdisciplinary teams work together completely to allow collaboration for assessment, planning, and intervention. Transdisciplinary teams blend boundaries in that one profession could assist with another profession for assessment and intervention; an example of this would be the SLP working on physical placement (sitting up), even though that would typically be addressed by a physical therapist. Interprofessional collaborative practice (IPCP) teams work very closely together through their dedication to collaborative assessment and treatment and include caregivers, the patient, and all professionals involved. Because working with someone with cognitive impairments may involve many areas of concern, using a teaming model is recommended.

During an assessment for intellectual or developmental disabilities, the clinician is going to want to assess different skills and areas. Use of nonsymbolic language (gestures, vocalizations), symbolic communication (signs, words), social interaction, spoken language, written language, oral motor skills, speech production, swallowing, and fluency are all areas that should be assessed. Patients will have varying abilities and no one way for assessing is recommended. If augmentative and alternative communication devices are used, that information will be needed. Determining if the patient is using the appropriate device should be evaluated. There are also standardized and nonstandardized test options. Standardized tests will give the clinician the ability to compare the client's skills with skills of other individuals. Nonstandardized test options will allow the clinician to tailor the assessment more specifically to the patient in order to assess function, strengths, and weaknesses.

Assessments for patients with dementia or other memory issues should include case history; recent/past medical history or status; cultural or linguistic background; review of auditory, visual, motor, cognitive and emotional status; interview with patient/family; as well as standardized and nonstandardized tests to determine communication, fluency, social, and swallowing abilities. Because dementia is considered progressive, a clinician should always be aware of a patient's changes in skills. When determining what standardized test(s) may be most beneficial, the clinician will want to make sure they are using an assessment tool that is appropriate for the patient's level. Some standardized assessment tools may be too difficult for a patient's current level. Giving an assessment in which a patient fails most all items is not helpful for the clinician to be able to appropriately diagnose the current level of functioning, nor be able to plan appropriate intervention.

An SLP will not be the one to diagnose the TBI, but he/she should be involved in the assessment of the patient. Traumatic brain injury assessments will follow closely the same assessment plan as for a patient with dementia. Screenings are typically conducted prior to a full evaluation. Case history and medical information will be vital for determining the appropriate testing protocol. Knowing a patient's hearing, visual, motor, emotional, cognitive, and social levels will also be vital. A clinician will want to know a patient's prior level of functioning. If a patient did not have certain skills or had strengths or weaknesses that had been determined prior to the TBI, a clinician may need to adjust the testing protocol. A clinician will determine what areas the patient is struggling with and in what contexts. Knowing this information will assist in the planning and addressing expectations of the patient. When assessing a patient with TBI, the clinician will need to assess the integrity of the patient's subsystems (respiration, phonation, etc.) (Traumatic Brain Injury, n.d.). Oral-motor abilities, speech motor planning, and swallowing will also need to be determined. Considerations during the assessment include presence of depression, side effects of medications, and existence of previous TBI. When completing the assessment, the clinician should be aware of the chance for motor deficits, sensory deficits, neurobehavioral deficits, and level of consciousness (Traumatic Brain Injury, n.d.). After certain types of brain injury, neurological recovery can occur for several months or longer (Traumatic Brain Injury, n.d.). Periodic assessments for patients with TBI is important.

Top 10 Terms

Intellectual disability

Developmental disability

Glasgow Coma Scale

Rancho Los Amigos Levels of Cognitive Functioning

Dementia

Traumatic brain injury

Nonsymbolic communication

Symbolic communication

Transdisciplinary team

Teaming model

Chapter Tips

1. Cognitive issues can be present across the life span.
2. Both standardized and nonstandardized assessment procedures are recommended in order to determine cognitive strengths/weaknesses.
3. Neurological recovery can occur for months or longer following a traumatic brain injury.

Activities

21-1. Read the following descriptions and determine if the description is more likely ID, TBI, or dementia:

_____ **1.** A 14-year-old female who is being brought to the clinic by family members who are most concerned with her ability to understand numbers and keep friends. It has been reported that she had to sit out of soccer for 2 weeks due to a concussion.

_____ **2.** A 64-year-old male who is at the clinic for an evaluation due to some concerns he has about his communication skills. During the interview, he mentions recently feeling depressed, having difficulty following conversations, cannot report what he ate for dinner last night, and repeats himself several times.

_____ **3.** A 9-year-old female who is functioning at a kindergarten level. She is just beginning to have letter recognition with some letters, has difficulty writing her name, has poor sequencing abilities, cannot follow two-step directions, and has no concept of time or sequencing.

_____ **4.** An 88-year-old male who has recently had a car accident. His verbal responses to questions are delayed and although he is able to say many words, the words do not make sense when put together to form thoughts.

_____ **5.** A 20-year-old male who is completing a certificate program through his high school. He hopes to transition to a community program where he will live and work in the community. He has some difficulty with planning, maintaining appropriate social interactions, making clear speech sounds, and expressing his wants/needs in a clear, concise manner.

_____ **6.** A 70-year-old female who trips and hits her head on the concrete driveway and loses consciousness for less than 5 min. She reports headaches and memory loss.

_____ **7.** An 18-month-old child who is showing some gross delays in speech/language. Medical history reveals child is in foster care and was taken from parents due to being shaken as a 4-month-old.

21-2. Read the following descriptions and determine, from the following list, what your next step would likely be (more than one answer may be appropriate).

    A. Read medical chart

    B. Obtain case history

    C. Interview patient/family/friends

    D. Collaborate with team

    E. Complete a screening

_____ **1.** You just completed a review of a medical chart for a patient who is going to be discharged from the hospital following a car wreck. Medical personnel have noticed no major concerns with regard to speech/language/swallowing but you were asked to complete "some testing" prior to discharge.

_____ **2.** You are scheduled to complete an evaluation in the clinic this morning. At this time, you only have a referral for a speech-language evaluation due to communication concerns for a 4-year-old.

_____ **3.** You have just completed an interview with the patient (a 76-year-old male). Based on the case history, the patient has had no new medical issues and his biggest concern was some recent swallowing issues. His daughter and wife accompanied him to the session, but they remained in the waiting room. Based on his inability to maintain topic of conversation, his delayed responses, his word-finding issues, and his repeating information, you are concerned with the additional communication problems and the accuracy of his report on his swallowing difficulties. He has given you permission to talk with his family.

_____ **4.** A nurse stops you in the hallway and lets you know that the doctor on call has just put in an order for an evaluation of the patient in room 246.

_____ **5.** You have reviewed the case history and referral information on a school-age client who has been receiving occupational therapy, physical therapy, and speech services, and has been receiving homebound education services due to the fragility of her medical condition. She recently moved to the area and is in need of a reevaluation due to IEP timelines and to determine a plan for services.

Answers to Activities

21–1.

1. TBI
2. Dementia
3. ID
4. TBI
5. ID
6. TBI
7. TBI/ID

21–2.

1. E
2. B
3. C

4. A
5. D

Wrap-Up

1. Complete some additional research on the Glasgow Coma Scale. Answer the following questions.

   What areas are assessed?

   _____
   _____

   How does a clinician assess those areas?

   _____
   _____
   _____
   _____
   _____
   _____
   _____
   _____
   _____
   _____

   How is the score interpreted?

   _____
   _____
   _____
   _____
   _____

   What are the ratings/what do they mean?

   _____
   _____

2. Complete some additional research on the Rancho Los Amigos Levels of Cognitive Functioning. Synthesize the information and put into your own words the description for each level.

Level 1: _____

Level 2: _____

Level 3: _____

Level 4: _____

_____
_____
_____

Level 5: _____
_____
_____
_____
_____
_____

Level 6: _____
_____
_____
_____
_____
_____

Level 7: _____
_____
_____
_____
_____
_____

Level 8: _____
_____
_____
_____
_____
_____

References

Dementia. (n.d.). Retrieved January 28, 2018, from https://www.asha.org/Practice-Portal/Clinical-Topics/Dementia/

Golper, L. A. (2010). *Medical speech-language pathology: A desk reference* (3rd ed.). Clifton Park, NY: Delmar.

Intellectual disability. (n.d.). Retrieved January 28, 2018, from https://www.asha.org/Practice-Portal/Clinical-Topics/Intellectual-Disability/

Shipley, K. G., & McAfee, J. G. (2016). *Assessment in speech-language pathology* (5th ed.). Boston, MA: Cengage Learning.

Traumatic brain injury in adults. (n.d.). Retrieved January 28, 2018, from https://www.asha.org/Practice-Portal/Clinical-Topics/Traumatic-Brain-Injury-in-Adults/

CHAPTER 22

Social Communication Assessment

Who

Social communication disorders (SCD) can occur at any age. Primarily, SCD assessments for children occur as differences are noticed when language skills begin developing; however, adults who have not been diagnosed previously and have a traumatic brain injury, stroke, or other medical condition such as brain tumors or Alzheimer's disease may also develop an SCD.

Different cultures have different expectations when communicating. When assessing for an SCD, it is important to keep in mind and be sensitive to the differences in cultures. For example, in some cultures eye contact is disrespectful; however, in America, eye contact is expected during conversations—yet, at the same time, staring is considered rude.

What

The American Speech-Language-Hearing Association (ASHA) defines social communication as "the use of language in social contexts" (Social communication disorder, n.d.). A SCD could be described as difficulty with social interactions, pragmatics, and/or social language. We use language in a variety of ways including maneuvering through conversations, using appropriate greetings, maintaining eye contact, and understanding or identifying emotions.

The following criterion for social (pragmatic) communication disorder is from the *Diagnostic and Statistical Manual of Mental Disorders, Fifth Edition* (DSM-5; American Psychiatric Association, 2013)

  A. Persistent difficulties in the social use of verbal and nonverbal communication as manifested by all of the following:

  1. Deficits in using communication for social purposes, such as greeting and sharing information, in a manner that is appropriate for social context.

  2. Impairment in the ability to change communication to match context or the needs of the listener, such as speaking differently in a classroom than on

a playground, talking differently to a child than to an adult, and avoiding use of overly formal language.

3. Difficulties following rules for conversation and storytelling, such as taking turns in conversation, rephrasing when misunderstood, and knowing how to use verbal and nonverbal signals to regulate interaction.

4. Difficulties understanding what is not explicitly stated (e.g., making inferences) and nonliteral or ambiguous meaning of language (e.g., idioms, humor, metaphors, multiple meanings that depend on the context for interpretation). (p. 47–49)

B. The deficits result in functional limitations in effective communication, social participation, social relationships, academic achievement, or occupational performance, individually or in combination.

C. The onset of the symptoms is in the early developmental period (but deficits may not fully manifest until social communication demands exceed limited capacities).

D. The symptoms are not attributable to another medical or neurological condition or to low abilities in the domains of word structure and grammar, and are not better explained by autism spectrum disorder, intellectual disability (intellectual developmental disorder), global developmental delay, or another mental disorder.

Keeping these statements from ASHA and the DSM-5 in mind, it is important to realize that assessing for SCDs requires authentic assessment. That is, the clinician must use a variety of resources such as observations in multiple settings if possible, parent questionnaires, interviews with caregivers, play assessment, communication analysis, and case history reports. In order to diagnose a SCD, the clinician must also keep cultural norms in mind. Different cultures have various expectations regarding social engagement during communication and clinicians should familiarize themselves with cultural norms as appropriate for each patient.

Disorders can range from mild to profound. Disorders are categorized by severity based on how the SCD impacts the life of a patient. It is important to think about educational, social, and work impacts for each patient. Various behaviors can impact one aspect of a patient's life tremendously, while not being a problem in other areas. For example, not recognizing emotions may not impact a child academically as much as it would keep him/her from making friends or potentially limiting future relationships.

Why

Social interactions are important. This is our ability to connect with others and feel included. Determining a patient's social abilities and weaknesses can assist in providing treatment options to allow him/her to be more involved in situations he/she will encounter on a daily basis.

When

Autism spectrum diagnoses are typically made in early childhood (toddler) or early school-age years. Research is increasing on early diagnosis and professionals are calling for diagnosis as early as possible in order to start intervention (Swain, Eadie, Prior, & Reilly, 2015). Often, things to look for are not what a child is doing but rather what a child is not doing. For example, a child who does not often respond to social requests (responding when someone calls his/her name) could be exhibiting some autistic behaviors. Concern can arise when a child does not point to convey a want/need or draw attention to something, does not use eye contact, does not engage in imaginative play, does not imitate actions of others (waving), among other things. When thinking about SCDs, a clinician should be watching for evidence of a lack of knowledge or use of the pragmatic aspects of language.

With adults, a clinician would be watching for a lack of social communication knowledge or use. Oftentimes, someone who experiences a right side stroke may lose the ability to assign emotional meaning to a conversation, may perseverate on topics, or may lose the ability to understand figurative language (idioms, similes, and/or irony). Sometimes a clinician may find that a person who experiences a right side stroke has difficulty with conversational turn taking.

All of these items discussed are difficult and perhaps even impossible to assess by using only a standard communication evaluation tool. It may be possible to utilize a checklist as part of a language assessment, but many of the social aspects of communication are better identified by observation and elicitation.

Where

As discussed earlier in this chapter, the best scenario is to use observations from a variety of settings. This allows the clinician to make better decisions on the pervasiveness of the social disorder. Often, children have a difficult time warming up to a clinician in a clinical setting and may respond very differently to adults than to peers. If an evaluation cannot take place across multiple settings, the clinician should be sure to utilize other professionals working with the patient or interviews with a variety of people involved in the patient's life.

How

Assessments could start with a screening that revealed some concerns or as part of a comprehensive speech/language assessment. Anytime a concern is noted through a screening, case history, or report, a full evaluation should be completed. Because hearing loss could cause behaviors that mimic a social language disorder, a hearing test should be completed to rule out hearing loss.

Knowing the norms for a person's age is very important when assessing for SCDs. If a clinician is unfamiliar with age norms, he/she may misdiagnose a problem or the lack of a problem. Age norms are typically established from birth to early school-age years. Social communication skills are developed by school age and do not change upon becoming geriatric, unless some other medical issue has developed (Alzheimer's disease, dementia,

TBI, hearing loss etc.); therefore, if an adult is experiencing issues that should have been developed or had been developed and are now lost, he/she could be considered disordered.

Case history is important as it can give you information and indications of behaviors or issues that you may not have the opportunity to see during an assessment session. Case history can also give you an idea of concomitant issues. SCDs can occur in isolation or in conjunction with other disorders. Case history information can also help direct the assessment process and provide the clinician with information on likes/dislikes and ways to better elicit certain behaviors.

There are checklists and forms that could be used during or prior to an assessment session that can allow caregivers to provide information on how a child typically responds. These forms are helpful in covering a broad array of topics related to social communication. In some instances, the forms or checklists serve as a type of screening form (Shipley & McAfee, 2016). The clinician could also complete the form/checklist with the parent/caregiver in order to expand on topics or areas that may need more explanation.

During the assessment, the clinician will want to observe the client's behavior as well as provide opportunities for the child to exhibit certain skills. Examples of things you may want to see is the skill of requesting (does the child point to the object, gesture if he/she wants it, verbally request it, etc.), joint attention (does he/she pay attention to an object that you are engaged with), pretend play, echolalia (repeating things heard using similar inflection/timing), and recognizing emotions. That is not an all-inclusive list, but as a clinician it is your responsibility to know what skills are appropriate for the client's age and how to set up an environment to allow the client to show you those skills. This is why one assessment session may not allow a clinician to know what a client is fully capable of and why multiple settings may help provide additional needed opportunities to assess the client's skills. Using a multidisciplinary team approach can be very beneficial when assessing for SCD. Members of other professions or other stakeholders patient's life can provide additional information or points of view that will allow for a broader picture of the patient's life, strengths, and weaknesses. For adults, it is often easy to elicit appropriate social behaviors through conversation as well as through providing pictures, which can help provide opportunities to evaluate the client's ability to recognize various emotions.

Analyzing conversational samples is another important tool that can be utilized. By recording conversation exchanges or having the client tell a story (either one he/she develops or perhaps by giving him/her a book of pictures in which he/she has to describe what is happening) and further analyzing that recording, the clinician can obtain additional information on the client's abilities. When analyzing communication samples for SCDs, the clinician will be looking for things such as the client's ability to predict, their ability to have typical conversation exchanges, their ability to transition, their reactions when change or complications are introduced, as well as other social aspects of communication.

Top 10 Terms

Social communication

Pragmatics

DSM-V

Autism

Joint attention

Echolalia

Pretend play

Asperger's syndrome

Nonverbal

Figurative language

Chapter Tips

1. SCDs are typically identified in toddlers/early school-age children; however, new research is allowing for earlier diagnosis, which is important for early intervention and communication success.
2. Elicitation of behaviors is often needed during an assessment.
3. Assessments involving multiple settings/professionals/caregivers will allow the clinician to make a more accurate diagnosis and develop a treatment plan.

Activities

22–1. Read the following scenarios and determine the areas that you would be concerned with or would like additional information about to determine if an SCD is present.

   A. An 18-month-old who babbles but does not use any words, does not establish eye contact, squeals for attention, reaches up to be picked up, and has no interest in looking in a mirror.

   _____
   _____
   _____
   _____

   B. A 3-year-old who does not use any greetings, does not use intonation, responds to name, does not use imaginative play, follows two-step directions, does not attend to items others are paying attention to, and relies heavily on gestures to get needs/wants met.

   _____
   _____
   _____
   _____

C. A 6-year-old who is described as a loner, uses primarily statements, can repeat movie lines verbatim, loves to talk about dinosaurs and numbers (is hard to redirect to other topics), cannot answer questions related to feelings in a story, and is impulsive.

D. An 82 year-old who recently experienced a right hemisphere stroke, can express wants/needs, loves to talk about her family (is difficult to have a conversation with about anything else), does not understand jokes, and does not pay attention to the emotions of others.

22–2. Determine three activities you would use to elicit certain behaviors for the following ages. Identify what you hope the activity will elicit.

A. A 2-year-old:

Activity 1: _____

Activity 2: _____

Activity 3: _____

B. A 7-year-old:

Activity 1: _____

Activity 2: _____

_____

_____

Activity 3: _____

_____

_____

C. A 76-year-old:

Activity 1: _____

_____

_____

Activity 2: _____

_____

_____

Activity 3: _____

_____

_____

Answers to Activities

22–1.

A. An 18-month-old who babbles but does not use any words, does not establish eye contact, squeals for attention, reaches up to be picked up, and has no interest in looking in a mirror.
- Not using words
- No eye contact
- Using squeals in the absence of words
- No interest in engaging with mirror play

B. A 3-year-old who does not use any greetings, does not use intonation, responds to name, does not use imaginative play, follows two-step directions, does not attend to items others are paying attention to, and relies heavily on gestures to get needs/wants met.
- Absence of greeting use
- Absence of intonation

- Not engaging in imaginative play
- No joint attention
- Relying on gestures in the absence of coupling with words

C. A 6-year-old who is described as a loner, uses primarily statements, can repeat movie lines verbatim, loves to talk about dinosaurs and numbers (is hard to redirect to other topics), cannot answer questions related to feelings in a story, and is impulsive.

- Lack of social relationships
- Not using questions
- Echolalia
- Topic perseveration
- Dictating conversation by perseveration
- Lack of emotional awareness of others
- Impulsive behaviors

D. An 82 year-old who recently experienced a right hemisphere stroke, can express wants/needs, loves to talk about her family (is difficult to have a conversation with about anything else), does not understand jokes, and does not pay attention to the emotions of others.

- Topic dominance/perseveration
- Lack of figurative language awareness/abilities
- Lack of emotional awareness of others

22–2.

A. A 2-year-old:

Activity 1: Put something of high desire out of reach.

You would do this to see what techniques the child would use to request the desired item.

Activity 2: Give the child something to play with; when the child is playing, take away the item and bring out something else.

You would do this to see if the child protests when something is taken away. You could also see if the child can transition to a new activity.

Activity 3: Start "crying" during the session when you were perfectly happy seconds before.

You would do this to determine if the child recognizes the emotion shift. Does the child offer sympathy or try to figure out what happened?

B. A 7-year-old:

Activity 1: Give the child a picture book and ask him/her to make up a story about the pictures.

You would do this to determine if the child uses prediction and can make a logical sequence of events.

Activity 2: Give the child a puzzle with a piece missing.

You would do this to determine what strategies the child would use to let you know the puzzle could not be completed as well as to assess their requesting skills if he/she requests or looks for the missing piece.

Activity 3: Have the child interpret pictures of kids expressing different emotions.

You would do this to determine if the child can accurately identify emotions. Using interpretation, you could also find out if he/she can assign expected causes of the emotion.

C. A 76-year-old:

Activity 1: Ask the client to tell you what he/she does in an average day.

You could do this to determine if he/she can give you normal sequences that would occur in a day.

Activity 2: Draw topics from a hat as conversation starters.

You could do this to allow for conversational analysis. This could help you determine if the client uses typical exchanges, can talk about various things, can ask questions related to and consistent within a topic, and use inflections when appropriate.

Activity 3: Use pictures of various scenes revealing different emotions and ask why he/she thinks the person is having that emotion.

You would do this to determine if the client can relate events to appropriate emotional responses. You could also ask the client what he/she could do in each of the situations to determine if he/she has the ability to make decisions that would be relevant to the situation described.

Wrap-Up

1. Compare and contrast two autism checklists. Were these for the same ages or different ages? What were the similarities/differences? What aspects did you like? What aspects would you change?

   Checklist #1 Name: _____

   Checklist #2 Name: _____

   Similarities of the checklists: _____

   _____

   _____

   _____

   _____

Differences between the checklists: _____

_____

_____

_____

Aspects you like/were helpful: _____

_____

_____

_____

_____

Aspects you would change: _____

_____

_____

_____

_____

2. Look online at either videos or resources that describe normal development with a focus on social development. Synthesize the information for the following ages and write a synopsis of what should be expected at each age.

   Birth to 6 months:

   _____

   _____

   _____

   _____

   _____

   _____

   6 to 12 months:

   _____

   _____

   _____

1 to 2 years:

2 to 3 years:

3 to 4 years:

4 to 5 years:

5 to 6 years:

References

American Psychiatric Association. (2013). *Diagnostic and statistical manual of mental disorders* (5th ed.). Arlington, VA: Author.

Shipley, K. G., & McAfee, J. G. (2016). *Assessment in speech-language pathology* (5th ed.). Boston, MA: Cengage Learning.

Social communication disorders. (n.d.). Retrieved January 28, 2018, from https://www.asha.org/Practice-Portal/Clinical-Topics/Social-Communication-Disorders-in-School-Age-Children/

Swain, N. R., Eadie, P. A., Prior, M. R., & Reilly, S. (2015). Assessing early communication skills at 12 months: A retrospective study of autism spectrum disorder. *International Journal of Language & Communication Disorders, 50*(4), 488–498.

CHAPTER 23

Communication Modalities

Who

Everyone uses multiple modalities to communicate. A person might wave good morning to the driver of the car passing by, say good morning to a friend, nod to an acquaintance, text a partner that he/she has arrived safely, or write good morning on the classroom whiteboard for all to see. Likewise, an individual who is deaf may use speech, gestures, facial expressions, sign language, or writing to communicate information depending on the needs of the situation. An individual with significant multiple impairments may vocalize, express with facial and body movements, utilize object cues, and "read" object-based experience books. Another individual may rely on a highly sophisticated computerized device, slow and labored speech, and typed/voice output material in daily communication situations. In an assessment to determine the best way to aid use of communication modalities, a team of professionals would be actively involved in evaluating the client's wants/preferences, needs, strengths, and communication limitations. This team makes recommendations for individual, specific augmentative and alternative communication (AAC) strategies and equipment and helps in their training and use. The speech-language clinician plays a critical role in this team process.

Individuals needing communication modalities assessments are those who require an augmentation (addition to) or an alternative (different) way to speak, listen, read, and/or write. There is a wide variety of individuals with disorders who benefit from the inclusion of AAC to support communication. A partial list of disorders that frequently contain an AAC component includes autism, aphasia, deaf/hearing impaired, blind/visually impaired, laryngectomy, cerebral palsy, Parkinson's disease, cognitive impairment, and apraxia. Individuals being assessed in communication modalities represent a wide range of ages, cultures, sensory needs, cognitive abilities, and sensory and motor abilities. The variety of disabilities and range of individual characteristics makes this an important topic to explore, but also makes this a difficult topic to master.

What

Central to many AAC evaluations is the question of what strategies would be most beneficial to recommend to this individual to enhance their communication abilities? Some AAC involves unaided help, requiring nothing beyond the person; while other AAC involves aided help, requiring an outside device or material. Gesturing or signing are considered unaided, while a speech output device, hearing aid, or picture system are considered aided method. AAC devices can take many forms and levels of technical involvement. Some AAC aided devices involve little or no technology (low tech), while others require a higher degree of technological involvement (high tech). Beyond their degree of technological involvement, devices vary in the demands placed on cognitive, motor, sensory, and linguistic systems. They also vary in the aspect of communication being addressed (speaking, listening, reading, and/or writing).

All of our evaluation procedures may come into play in the AAC assessment. Identifying the aided or unaided system and high or low tech device to recommend will likely include:

1. interviews and questionnaires completed by the client, family, and others who interact with the client regularly;
2. formal standardized testing of areas such as cognitive, speech, and language/literacy abilities;
3. observation of current communication, sensory, and cognitive functioning across settings and partners;
4. structured interaction to test trial use of varied AAC device types and materials; and
5. dynamic procedures to identify effective teaching strategies.

Each of these procedures warrants a closer examination.

Interviews and questionnaires are an important part of the process. A variety of components needs to be addressed in the interview or through questionnaires. Clients' and families' wants, needs, and wishes as well as current levels of functioning and projected expectations of future needs provide the big picture framework for the assessment. Lawrence (2017) noted that in her many years of experience as a speech-language pathologist (SLP) specializing in AAC, client and family input during the assessment process makes an impact on later success and generalization of the selected AAC system. More definition is added to the big picture with information obtained through exploring current content, form and use of language and literacy, intelligibility of speech, sensory abilities in vision and hearing, motor facility, and behavioral factors. A detailed, fine-grained depiction is also needed. Specifics on which vocabulary words are used and needed; what words can be understood by listeners; precise visual acuity and function of vision in scanning and tracking; hearing acuity and functional use of the auditory signal; extent, accuracy, and consistency of specified body part movements; and response time, alertness, and energy level are some of the many details the clinician needs to obtain.

Standardized testing is useful in specifying the current level of functioning and comparing the individual's performance to that of his/her peers. However, the fact that the need for an AAC device is being considered implies that the individual's current system of communication needs to be augmented or an alternative means provided in order for the person to be a more successful communicator. There is no cognitive, physical, language, or literacy prerequisite level or cut off that indicates whether an individual would benefit from AAC help while another would not.

Observation of the individual in communication situations, preferably across typical partners and settings, is essential as it allows the evaluator to put the information provided in the interviews, questionnaires, and test performance into perspective. The assessment process often segments communication into components so one can get an understanding of each component. However, the components do not operate in isolation from each other; rather, in a holistic fashion. It is crucial to an evaluation that typical communication situations be examined.

Structured interactions promote a trial of exemplar AAC devices and materials to identify strengths and weaknesses of various systems for the individual client. An AAC assessment team will likely have a selection of devices and materials for trial purposes. State-wide, federally funded assistive technology resource centers (ATRC) will loan devices for trial use or manufacturers may provide short-term loaner devices for individuals to try.

When recommending the appropriate AAC system, the team must also consider effective strategies for teaching an individual to use his/her system. Dynamic assessment should identify the most promising method(s) for training with the system. Instruction, cueing hierarchies, demonstration, guided practice, hand-under-hand prompts, and both client and partner communication via devices are some of the possible strategies for learning that could be considered. Dynamic assessment can also provide an indication of readiness to learn specific material for young children who use AAC (Binger, Kent-Walsh, & King, 2017).

Why

An AAC recommendation is about developing or purchasing an AAC device that will best work for the individual, and avoiding developing or purchasing an AAC device and then attempting to make it work. The unprecedented access of AAC devices via the internet can result in getting the horse before the cart or selecting the device before a thorough evaluation has been performed. This can result in undermining the potential an appropriate AAC device may have or purchasing indiscriminately and wasting limited time and resources. Keeping up with the rapid advances in the technology in this area is daunting.

When

Multimodality assessment is a specialized, purpose-driven assessment. It is performed when a need for alternative or augmentative means are being considered to improve an individual's communication system.

Where

There is no one place where assessment must or should occur. Parts of the assessment are best done in one-on-one assessment/interviewing situations, while other parts are best in a naturalistic setting.

How

One truth in AAC assessment is that it should never be done in isolation. This should always be a team process that involves clients, family members, and multiple professionals. Several types of team organization have been described over the years beginning with multidisciplinary teams (which involve individual assessments by professionals merged together); next, interdisciplinary teams (which include an increased role for client and family members); then, transdisciplinary teams (which embrace shared assessment time and increased professional role release); and, most recently, interprofessional collaborative practice (IPCP; which requires strong commitment to both team structure and collaborative practices from assessment through treatment) (Ogletree et al., 2017; Sylverster, Ogletree, & Lunnen, 2017).

Top 10 Terms

Aided
Assistive technology resource center (ATRC)
Augmentative and alternative communication (AAC)
High tech
Interdisciplinary team
Interprofessional collaborative practice (IPCP)
Low tech
Multidisciplinary team
Transdisciplinary team
Unaided

Chapter Tips

1. Effective AAC use necessitates the involvement and often training of those who will be interacting with and supporting the user, as well as programing and maintaining the device or materials. Once a device is obtained, the work has just begun. Devices must be monitored, modified, and reassessed as the client's wants/preferences, needs, strengths, and limitations change. This is true for all AAC users but is most obvious in individuals with a progressive disorder. Always think of AAC assessment as ongoing.

2. AAC can be important at any age. Make sure your assessment and recommendations are adapted to meet the age of your client.

3. Consideration of receptive and expressive components are important. Some systems like partial object systems can serve both a receptive function (such as presenting a spoon to indicate meal time is next), and an expressive function (such as having the spoon available so the child can select it to indicate he/she is hungry). Other systems like a computer-generated voice output system are used for nonverbal individuals to expressively "voice" his/her message.

Activities

23–1. Identify if each of the following statements represents aided or unaided communication; record your answer in the space provided before the example. Next, identify if there is an AAC device described in the statement and whether it is high tech or low tech; record your answer in the space provided after the example.

1. _____ Teacher reported that Perry had no way to get her attention in the classroom until a signaling switch was introduced. He pushes the large switch to activate the voice output signal that says "Help please." _____

2. _____ Mr. Smith likes to have conversations about his grandchildren but cannot remember their names unless prompted with a photograph. He has a conversation book that is organized by topics and has appropriate photos and names that he uses to initiate conversations. _____

3. _____ Regina's team has initiated using a Plexiglas divider for her to make a visual choice (eye gaze) between pictures placed on the four quadrants of the board. _____

4. _____ Finnegan has limited visual acuity and uses prerecorded textbooks. _____

5. _____ Mrs. Asher is an active communication partner who relies on gestures to get her often unintelligible utterance across to her listener. _____

6. _____ Philippi, who has significant visual and hearing impairments, enjoyed rereading object-based experience books developed by the teacher or therapist to reflect on past activities. _____

7. _____ Ben has been using a picture exchange system that allows him to request wants and needs through selection of available pictures. _____

8. _____ Nurses provide hospital patients, who are not able to speak, with a laminated card for selecting degree of pain, site of pain, and yes/no responses. _____

9. _____ Maria can now be an active participant in her classroom morning circle time routine. She uses a nine choice device that is programed with the items from the morning circle time routine. _____

10. _____ An iPad with a purchased app allowed Oliver to make requests, give comments, or ask questions of those around him. He especially liked the fact that the voice sounded like a young male. _____

23–2. For each of the following assessment descriptions, identify the team structure described as multidisciplinary assessment, interdisciplinary assessment, transdisciplinary assessment, or interprofessional collaborative practice.

1. A case coordinator facilitated the joint assessment time where one professional interacted with the client following the prior plan/directions developed with the other team members (including the client's family as a team member). These team members observed the interaction, making notes during the joint observation, and met as a team afterward to develop the integrated report and recommendations. _____

2. The SLP, teacher, physical therapist, and vision specialist each evaluated the child at a separate time within a month. The four sets of information were combined into one report and a set of recommendations that were shared with the parent. _____

3. A case manager established an ongoing team of professionals working alongside the family to develop integrated recommendations including cotreatment options. The International Classification of Functioning, Disability and Health (World Health Organization, 2001) was used as a common system to integrate the varied professional jargon and develop joint assessment and remediation recommendations. _____

4. The SLP, teacher, psychologist, and reading teacher each evaluated the child at a separate time within a month. The parents were invited to attend each assessment and asked to provide goals they would like addressed. All the input and information was combined into one report and set of recommendations. _____

Answers to Activities

23–1.

First Blank	Second Blank
1. aided	high tech
2. aided	low tech
3. aided	low tech
4. aided	high tech

5. unaided	NA
6. aided	low tech
7. aided	low tech
8. aided	low tech
9. aided	high tech
10. aided	high tech

23-2.

1. transdisciplinary assessment
2. multidisciplinary assessment
3. interprofessional collaborative practice
4. interdisciplinary assessment

Wrap-Up

1. All states have federally supported assistive technology resource centers (ATRC). Locate the ATRC near where you hope to practice after graduation. List the location and the mission of your ATRC.

    Location:

    Mission:

2. The authors listed several disorders that frequently utilize an AAC component including autism, aphasia, deaf/hearing impaired, blind/visually impaired, laryngectomy, cerebral palsy, Parkinson's disease, cognitive impairment, and apraxia. Compare and contrast the likely AAC needs of two disorders from the list.

3. The communication needs of an adult client differ from the communication needs of a school-aged client. List three likely adult communication needs and three likely child communication needs for an AAC device.

   Common adult communication needs:

   Common child communication needs:

4. What might you say or do to help a client or family member who is reluctant to consider using AAC as a viable option?

References

Binger, C., Kent-Walsh, J., & King, M. (2017). Dynamic assessment for 3- and 4-year-old children who use augmentative and alternative communication: Evaluating expressive syntax. *Journal of Speech, Language, and Hearing Research, 60*, 1946–1958.

Lawrence, L. J. (2017). Tapping into the "augmentative" of AAC. *The ASHA Leader, 22*, 2, 38–39.

Ogletree, B. T., Brady, N., Bruce, S., Dean, E., Romski, M., Sylvester, L., & Westling, D. (2017). Mary's case: An illustration of interprofessional collaborative practice for a child with severe disabilities. *American Journal of Speech-Language Pathology, 26*, 217–226.

Sylverster, L., Ogletree, B. T., & Lunnen, K. (2017). Cotreatment as a vehicle for interprofessional collaborative practice: Physical therapist and speech-language pathologists collaborating in the care of children with severe disabilities. *American Journal of Speech-Language Pathology, 26*, 206–216.

World Health Organization. (2001). *International classification of functioning, disability and health (IFC)*. Geneva, Switzerland: World Health Organization.

CHAPTER 24

Final Thoughts

Who

This final chapter is about you and what you know. It is provided to help organize and integrate the material presented in the previous 23 chapters, to expand on some of your basic knowledge, and to provide an opportunity to apply what you have learned. Completing this book has hopefully aided in you becoming a more knowledgeable and, ultimately, an autonomous diagnostic clinician. Autonomy in the field of speech-language pathology is critical; it allows clinicians to make independent decisions on how best to assess and remediate their clients. As a student clinician, you are not autonomous but rather practicing as directed by your clinical supervisor.

This final chapter is directed at allowing you to demonstrate the knowledge you have acquired to develop diagnostic plans for clients across the nine disorder categories previously described as a step in the process of becoming an independent speech-language pathologist (SLP). The format of this chapter is different from previous chapters in several ways. Each of the following sections will require you to complete one or more charts. A corresponding answer chart to use as comparison is provided in the Answers to Charts section. These answer charts are not *the* right answer but rather *a* right answer. Seeing where/how you differ from the answer key should motivate you to consider other answers, to explore discrepancies between your answers and the key, and, ultimately, to return to the text for reexamination of the issues in question. The Top 10 Terms section will require you to analyze terms from the book by asking you to compare and contrast pairs of related terms.

To integrate standardized tests with the age of the normative sample, Table 24–1 provides a chart listing common standardized tests used in speech-language therapy as well as space for you to fill in up to five additional tests. Identify the age the test is normed for—preschool children: age 0 to 3; school-aged children: age 3 to 13; adolescents: age 13 to 18; or adult: age 18 and older. You can use any sources to locate this age data.

Table 24–1. Chart Listing Common Standardized Tests and Appropriate Ages

Standardized Test/Author(s)	Preschool Children	School-Aged Children	Adolescents	Adults
Western Aphasia Battery-Revised; WAB-R (Kertesz, 2007)				
Test of Language Development-Primary, Fourth Edition; TOLD-P:4 (Newcomer & Hammill, 2008)				
Preschool Language Scales, Fifth Edition; PLS-5 (Zimmerman, Steiner, & Pond, 2011)				
Diagnostic Evaluation of Articulation and Phonology; DEAP (Dodd, Hua, Crosbie, Holm, & Ozanne, 2006)				
Cognitive Linguistic Quick Test-Plus; CLQT+ (Helm-Estabrooks, 2001)				
Clinical Evaluation of Language Fundamentals, Fifth Edition; CELF-5 (Wiig, Semel, & Secord, 2013)				
Oral and Written Language Scales, Second Edition; OWLS-II (Carrow-Wollfork, 2011)				
Clinical Assessment of Articulation and Phonological, Second Edition; CAAP-2 (Secord & Donohue, 2013)				
Comprehensive Assessment of Spoken Language, Second Edition; CASL-2 (Carrow-Woolfolk, 2017)				
Peabody Picture Vocabulary Test, Fourth Edition; PPVT-4 (Dunn & Dunn, 2007)				
Goldman-Fristoe Test of Articulation, Third Edition; GFTA-3 (Goldman & Fristoe, 2015)				

What

The integration of form and procedure is needed when planning any assessment. Four kinds of common evaluation types have been described in Chapter 10 including initial evaluations, ongoing data collection, progress/reevaluations, and final/dismissal evaluations. Within each kind of evaluation is one or more common procedure that can be used to gather information. The common procedures considered in Table 24–2 include interview(s), hearing screening, oral peripheral examination, standardized test(s), observation, structured interaction(s), and dynamic assessment. Use this chart to rate how likely it is you would use the procedures presented in the first column in each type of evaluation using a 3-point scale (1 = very likely to collect; 2 = may collect; 3 = unlikely to collect). Make comments in the box to help clarify your rating.

Table 24–2. Chart Rating How Likely It Is You Would Use the Procedures Presented in Column 1 in Each Type of Evaluation Using a 3-Point Scale (1 = very likely to collect; 2 = may collect; 3 = unlikely to collect)

Procedure	Initial Evaluations	Ongoing Data Collection	Reevaluations	Dismissal Evaluations
Interview(s)				
Hearing Screening				
Oral Peripheral Examination				
Standardized Test(s)				
Observation				
Structured Interaction(s)				
Dynamic Assessment				

Why

Everything we do in an evaluation is done for a purpose. The big questions a clinician would answer through an assessment were addressed throughout the chapters in this book. What you are asked to explain in Table 24–3 are some of the subtler behaviors a clinician might exhibit in an assessment. Column 1 lists behaviors a clinician might exhibit; use column 2 to state a possible reasoning behind each behavior.

Table 24–3. Chart Explaining Behaviors a Clinician Might Exhibit in an Assessment and Possible Reasoning Behind These Behaviors

What Was Asked/Done	Why It Was Asked/Done and Possible Reasoning
Ask for parent to sign a consent form.	
Describe the test or procedure in the report (not just give the name of test).	
Ask the client why he/she came today (even a child).	
Fill out the test form completely.	
Screen hearing even when no hearing loss is reported.	
Gather baseline information.	
Make referrals.	
Always engage in or observe actual conversation.	
Proofed for content, spelling, and grammar in every written document.	
Included the highest degree obtained and "CCC-Speech" with the signature on the report.	

When

The integration of time and procedure used will vary depending on factors such as reason for the assessment, age of the client, and disorder area(s) of focus. For this integration exercise, you have 2 hrs (120 mins) to complete an initial assessment at a university-run clinic for Sally, a 4;6-year-old female, referred by her pediatrician for a speech and language evaluation due to delays in language and unintelligible speech. Use Table 24–4 to identify how your time will be spent (in 15-min time blocks) by noting, in column 2, the procedure or tasks of focus at for each time block. A procedure may run for more than one block of time. In column 2, also note your rationale for the order you are suggesting.

Table 24–4. Chart Identifying How You Would Divide Your Time (in 15-min Time Blocks) in an Initial Assessment. Note the Procedure or Tasks of Focus for Each Time Block

Time	Procedure
0–15 min	
16–30 min	
31–45 min	
46–60 min	
61–75 min	
76–90 min	
91–105 min	
116–120 min	

Where

As speech clinicians, we serve individuals in a variety of places. According to ASHA (n.d.), 56% of ASHA-certified clinicians are employed in educational settings (early intervention, preschool, K–12 schools, and colleges and universities), 39% in health care settings (nonresidential health care facilities, hospitals, and residential health care facilities), and 19% in full-time or part-time private practices. There is overlap between where a specific client might be served. The chart in Table 24–5 requires you to identify one or more places where an assessment would be conducted given a specific client description. Please be as specific as you can when identifying likely facilities (i.e., preschool or hospital) where the assessment would occur. The three blank rows are for you to describe a client and then identify the likely site of assessment.

Table 24–5. Chart Identifying One or More Places Where an Assessment Would Be Conducted Given a Specific Client Description

Description of Client	Education: Early Intervention, Preschool, K–12, or Colleges/ Universities	Health Care: Nonresidential, Residential, or Hospital	Private Practice: Single Person, Small Practice, or Large Practice
Paul Golden, a 67-year-old male Vietnam veteran, is being evaluated for			

continues

Table 24–5. (*continued*)

Description of Client	Education: Early Intervention, Preschool, K–12, or Colleges/ Universities	Health Care: Nonresidential, Residential, or Hospital	Private Practice: Single Person, Small Practice, or Large Practice
language abilities following a stroke with an onset of 1 day.			
Candy Griffen, a 7-year-old female, is being assessed by an outside agency in order to provide information for a due process hearing from the school.			
Eddie Worth, a 2;4-year-old male, is being referred for suspected autism.			
Holly Fant, a 20-year-old female with a significant cognitive delay and extended school services, is being reevaluated to update goals and objectives.			
Kim Lou, a 30-year-old male physician, is seeking assessment of his articulation to improve his communication skills with clients (note, this is not a disorder but a choice to obtain modification of a difference).			

How

Forethought and planning prior to an assessment is an important part of the process. Tables 24–6 through 24–15 provide an outline chart of information you should consider before presenting your supervisor with your plan for an initial assessment. Complete one chart for each of the nine disorder areas as though you are planning your first diagnostic with a potential client in this specific diagnostic category. Begin by reading the intake information in the first row and then proceed to answer each question in column 1 to help prepare you for your planning meeting with your diagnostic supervisor. The answer example charts were provided by students in the graduate Communication Sciences and Disorders program at Western Carolina University.

Table 24–6. Outline of the Information You Should Consider Before Presenting Your Supervisor With Your Plan for an Initial Assessment of a Speech Sound Disorder

Questions to Consider	Answer
Please summarize the intake information from this client (you can make up the specifics of the case you will explore).	10-year-old male. Trouble with /r/ words.
What diagnostic questions are you planning to address?	
What are three case-specific questions you will ask in the interview?	
What standardized test(s) do you plan to administer? Why these?	
Describe the informal assessment activities you are planning.	

continues

Table 24–6. (*continued*)

Questions to Consider	Answer
What three specific characteristics do you plan to make note of in an observation time?	
How will you determine recommendations for therapy?	
What might be +/– prognostic factors you are going to consider?	
How do you plan to get ready to perform this diagnostic (day before, day of, and day following the diagnostic)?	

Table 24–7. Outline of the Information You Should Consider Before Presenting Your Supervisor With Your Plan for an Initial Assessment of a Voice Disorder

Questions to Consider	Answer
Please summarize the intake information from this client (you can make up the specifics of the case you will explore).	The client is a 30-year-old who works as a middle school music teacher and teaches piano and private singing lessons as a side job. Per patient report, she drinks a lot of caffeine (at least four cups per day). She reports rough and breathy voicing as well as pitch breaks, and complains of a sore throat.

continues

Table 24–7. (*continued*)

Questions to Consider	Answer
What diagnostic questions are you planning to address?	
What are three case-specific questions you will ask in the interview?	
What standardized test(s) do you plan to administer? Why these?	
Describe the informal assessment activities you are planning.	
What three specific characteristics do you plan to make note of in an observation time?	
How will you determine recommendations for therapy?	
What might be +/− prognostic factors you are going to consider?	
How do you plan to get ready to perform this diagnostic (day before, day of, and day following the diagnostic)?	

Table 24–8. Outline of the Information You Should Consider Before Presenting Your Supervisor With Your Plan for an Initial Assessment of a Fluency Disorder

Questions to Consider	Answer
Please summarize the intake information from this client (you can make up the specifics of the case you will explore).	Mike is an intelligent and thoughtful 9-year-old boy whose family has recently moved to the area. He has just transferred to your school and has been referred to you. At his previous school, Mike received speech therapy targeting his stutter. His mother reportedly stuttered as a child, but spontaneously recovered in high school. His mother also stated that she is concerned about Mike making friends at his new school due to his insecurities about his stutter. It was reported that Mike had pressure equalization (P.E.) tubes placed in his ears at age 2, but other than that, medical history is unremarkable.
What diagnostic questions are you planning to address?	
What are three case-specific questions you will ask in the interview?	
What standardized test(s) do you plan to administer? Why these?	
Describe the informal assessment activities you are planning.	

continues

Table 24–8. (*continued*)

Questions to Consider	Answer
What three specific characteristics do you plan to make note of in an observation time?	
How will you determine recommendations for therapy?	
What might be +/– prognostic factors you are going to consider?	
How do you plan to get ready to perform this diagnostic (day before, day of, and day following the diagnostic)?	

Table 24–9. Outline of the Information You Should Consider Before Presenting Your Supervisor With Your Plan for an Initial Assessment of a Language/Literacy Disorder in Children/Adolescents

Questions to Consider	Answer
Please summarize the intake information from this client (you can make up the specifics of the case you will explore).	The client, Kelsey, is a 7-year; 4-month-old female whose first language is English. She was referred to the school SLP by her first grade teacher. Her teacher reports that Kelsey often "stares blankly" when asked a direct question and gives unrelated answers or declines answering. The teacher also stated that Kelsey has difficulty following whole-class directions and has trouble remembering vocabulary from the content taught in class from one day to the next. The short questionnaire sent home to Kelsey's parents revealed that she attended private preschool for 2 years because they "thought she just wasn't quite ready for kindergarten." Kelsey passed her hearing screening at the beginning of the year. Both her teacher and her parents report that Kelsey is a happy, curious girl. Her teacher reports that she is very timid around her peers except for two close friends in class.
What diagnostic questions are you planning to address?	
What are three case-specific questions you will ask in the interview?	
What standardized test(s) do you plan to administer? Why these?	

continues

Table 24–9. (continued)

Questions to Consider	Answer
Describe the informal assessment activities you are planning.	
What three specific characteristics do you plan to make note of in an observation time?	
How will you determine recommendations for therapy?	
What might be +/− prognostic factors you are going to consider?	
How do you plan to get ready to perform this diagnostic (day before, day of, and day following the diagnostic)?	

Table 24–10. Outline of the Information You Should Consider Before Presenting Your Supervisor With Your Plan for an Initial Assessment of a Language Disorder in Adults

Questions to Consider	Answer
Please summarize the intake information from this client (you can make up the specifics of the case you will explore).	The client is a 61-year-old male who came into the outpatient clinic complaining of difficulties with his speech. His wife mentioned that he had a stroke 6 months ago caused by occlusion to the middle cerebral artery of the inferior posterior frontal lobe of the left hemisphere. He is married and has two children who are in college. The wife is concerned about his speaking skills which sound telegraphic. His speaking is effortful and labored and composed of many misarticulations.
What diagnostic questions are you planning to address?	
What are three case-specific questions you will ask in the interview?	
What standardized test(s) do you plan to administer? Why these?	
Describe the informal assessment activities you are planning.	
What three specific characteristics do you plan to make note of in an observation time?	

continues

Table 24–10. (continued)

Questions to Consider	Answer
How will you determine recommendations for therapy?	
What might be +/– prognostic factors you are going to consider?	
How do you plan to get ready to perform this diagnostic (day before, day of, and day following the diagnostic)?	

Table 24–11. Outline of the Information You Should Consider Before Presenting Your Supervisor With Your Plan for an Initial Assessment of a Cognitive Disorder

Questions to Consider	Answer
Please summarize the intake information from this client (you can make up the specifics of the case you will explore).	Client is a 27-year-old female with a traumatic brain injury (TBI) following a motor vehicle accident. She was hospitalized at WakeMed Hospital for 3 months and received intensive inpatient rehabilitation while there. The client now lives at home with her mother and younger sister. Her family reported that the client is easily distracted both in conversation and while reading. The client has difficulty recalling information shortly after it is delivered. She also has poor orientation skills.

continues

Table 24–11. (continued)

Questions to Consider	Answer
What diagnostic questions are you planning to address?	
What are three case-specific questions you will ask in the interview?	
What standardized test(s) do you plan to administer? Why these?	
Describe the informal assessment activities you are planning.	
What three specific characteristics do you plan to make note of in an observation time?	
How will you determine recommendations for therapy?	
What might be +/– prognostic factors you are going to consider?	
How do you plan to get ready to perform this diagnostic (day before, day of, and day following the diagnostic)?	

Table 24–12. Outline of the Information You Should Consider Before Presenting Your Supervisor With Your Plan for an Initial Assessment of a Social Communication Disorder

Questions to Consider	Answer
Please summarize the intake information from this client (you can make up the specifics of the case you will explore).	The client moved to a new school district at the beginning of the previous school year. He was receiving therapy at his previous school and has an active IEP targeting receptive and expressive language skills. His second grade teacher has requested that he be evaluated for a possible social communication disorder. His teacher noted that he seems to have difficulty interacting with other classmates appropriately and expresses his frustration in a negative way, often screaming at his peers and having difficulty taking the perspective of others when he is upset. No case history or other information was transferred with the student to the new school, just the objectives his previous SLP was targeting in therapy.
What diagnostic questions are you planning to address?	
What are three case-specific questions you will ask in the interview?	
What standardized test(s) do you plan to administer? Why these?	
Describe the informal assessment activities you are planning.	

continues

Table 24–12. (continued)

Questions to Consider	Answer
What three specific characteristics do you plan to make note of in an observation time	
How will you determine recommendations for therapy?	
What might be +/– prognostic factors you are going to consider?	
How do you plan to get ready to perform this diagnostic (day before, day of, and day following the diagnostic)?	

Table 24–13. Outline of the Information You Should Consider Before Presenting Your Supervisor With Your Plan for an Initial Assessment of a Communication Modality Disorder

Questions to Consider	Answer
Please summarize the intake information from this client (you can make up the specifics of the case you will explore).	This client is a child of 5 years who has cerebral palsy and has a diagnosis of severe dysarthria; some apraxic-like groping is present. Functionally, the child has age-appropriate receptive language and minimal expressive language with average pragmatic skills. The child is able to complete most age-appropriate gross motor movements independently, but has difficulty with fine motor skills due to incoordination and some weakness. This client attends school in a regular classroom and has an aid to assist. The child's parents aren't happy with the progress their child has made despite speech therapy since the age of 3 and want to try a speech generation device.
What diagnostic questions are you planning to address?	
What are three case-specific questions you will ask in the interview?	
What standardized test(s) do you plan to administer? Why these?	
Describe the informal assessment activities you are planning.	

continues

Table 24–13. (*continued*)

Questions to Consider	Answer
What three specific characteristics do you plan to make note of in an observation time?	
How will you determine recommendations for therapy?	
What might be +/– prognostic factors you are going to consider?	
How do you plan to get ready to perform this diagnostic (day before, day of, and day following the diagnostic)?	

Table 24–14. Outline of the Information You Should Consider Before Presenting Your Supervisor With Your Plan for an Initial Assessment of an Audiology Disorder

Questions to Consider	Answer
Please summarize the intake information from this client (you can make up the specifics of the case you will explore).	Mr. Jones is a 59-year-old male who is complaining of difficulty hearing. He reported that his right ear is his "good ear." He first noticed the hearing loss around five years ago, and it has progressively worsened. As a young child, Mr. Jones had two ear infections. He has never had a serious head injury or ear surgery. Mr. Jones first consulted his primary care physician about his difficulty hearing 2 weeks ago; he was given a referral to an audiologist for a complete hearing assessment. Mr. Jones does not have a family history of hearing loss. He also complains of hearing ringing in his ears when no noise is present, but does not report feelings of dizziness. He does not have a history of serious illnesses, and is not currently taking any medications. Mr. Jones is presently employed. He works in construction as a foreman. He reports difficulty understanding speech both on the job and at home.
What diagnostic questions are you planning to address?	
What are three case-specific questions you will ask in the interview?	
What standardized test(s) do you plan to administer? Why these?	

continues

Table 24–14. (continued)

Questions to Consider	Answer
Describe the informal assessment activities you are planning.	
What three specific characteristics do you plan to make note of in an observation time?	
How will you determine recommendations for therapy?	
What might be +/– prognostic factors you are going to consider?	
How do you plan to get ready to perform this diagnostic (day before, day of, and day following the diagnostic)?	

Table 24–15. Swallowing Disorder Example (R. A. Cox, Personal Communication, October 23, 2017). Modifications to Include Citations Were Added.

Questions to Consider	Answer
Please summarize the intake information from this client (you can make up the specifics of the case you will explore).	Amy is a 52-year-old female who is happily married with two children. On Mondays and Wednesdays, she serves at a local church where she is the secretary. For the past 6 months, she has noticed that her body is changing. Both her and her family have noticed the following: loss of coordination, weak muscles, vocal pitch changes, slurred speech, muscle cramping, periods of uncontrollable laughing and crying, breathing difficulties, and trouble walking long distances. Amy's physician referred her to a neurologist where she received the diagnosis of amyotrophic lateral sclerosis (ALS). After receiving the diagnosis, a couple weeks later she began noticing difficulties swallowing. Not only does she have difficulties eating and drinking, but sometimes, especially late at night, she has trouble swallowing. In addition, her husband reported that she consistently drools. Her neurologist referred her to see a SLP to have a swallowing evaluation. Two weeks before her speech therapy appointment, Amy was diagnosed with pneumonia and is currently taking antibiotics.
What diagnostic questions are you planning to address?	
What are three case-specific questions you will ask in the interview?	
What standardized test(s) do you plan to administer? Why these?	

continues

Table 24–15. (continued)

Questions to Consider	Answer
Describe the informal assessment activities you are planning.	
What three specific characteristics do you plan to make note of in an observation time?	
How will you determine recommendations for therapy?	
What might be +/– prognostic factors you are going to consider?	
How do you plan to get ready to perform this diagnostic (day before, day of, and day following the diagnostic)?	

Top 10 Terms

Compare and contrast the following 10 sets of terms:

    Assessment versus evaluation:

    _____

    _____

    Basal versus ceiling:

    _____

    _____

Diagnostic report versus SOAP note writing:

Open questions versus closed questions:

Progress report versus final report:

Screening versus diagnostic testing:

Standardized testing versus dynamic assessment:

Structure versus function of oral mechanism:

Trial item versus test item:

ICD-10 codes versus CPT codes:

Chapter Tips

1. You do your client a disservice if you do not know about assessment. Remember to constantly be in tune with the questions you are trying to answer and the variety of methods you can use to obtain relevant information.
2. Presence of data is not enough. You must be able to interpret and describe the information to others in both oral and written formats.
3. Learning how best to do diagnostics is a lifelong process. Keep learning!

Wrap-Up

Answers to Charts

Answer Who Chart

Table 24–16. Chart Listing Common Standardized Tests and Appropriate Ages

Standardized Test/Author(s)	Preschool Children	School-Aged Children	Adolescents	Adults
Western Aphasia Battery-Revised; WAB-R (Kertesz, 2007)			18–89	18–89
Test of Language Development, Fourth Edition; TOLD-P:4 (Newcomer & Hammill, 2008)	4–8;10	4–8;10		
Preschool Language Scales, Fifth Edition; PLS-5 (Zimmerman, Steiner, & Pond, 2011)	Birth–7;11	Birth–7;11		
Diagnostic Evaluation of Articulation and Phonology; DEAP (Dodd, Hua, Crosbie, Holm, & Ozanne, 2006)	3;0–8;11	3;0–8;11		
Cognitive Linguistic Quick Test-Plus; CLQT + (Helm-Estabrooks, 2001)			18–89	18–89

continues

Table 24–16. (continued)

Standardized Test/Author(s)	Preschool Children	School-Aged Children	Adolescents	Adults
Clinical Evaluation of Language Fundamentals, Fifth Edition; CELF-5 (Wiig, Semel, & Secord, 2013)		5;0–21;11	5;0–21;11	
Oral and Written Language Scales, Second Edition; OWLS-II (Carrow-Wollfork, 2011)	3–21:11	3–21:11	3–21;11	3–21;11
Clinical Assessment of Articulation and Phonological, Second Edition; CAAP-2 (Secord & Donohue, 2013)	2;6–11;11	2;6–11;11		
Comprehensive Assessment of Spoken Language, Second Edition; CASL-2 (Carrow-Woolfolk, 2017)	3–21;11	3–21;11	3–21;11	3–21;11
Peabody Picture Vocabulary Test, Fourth Edition; PPVT-4 (Dunn & Dunn, 2007)	2;6–90+	2;6–90+	2;6–90+	2;6–90+
Goldman-Fristoe Test of Articulation, Third Edition; GFTA-3 (Goldman & Fristoe, 2015)	2–21;11	2–21;11	2–21;11	2–21;11

What Chart

Table 24–17. Chart Rating How Likely It Is You Would Use the Procedures Presented in Column 1 in Each Type of Evaluation Using a 3-Point Scale (1 = very likely to collect; 2 = may collect; 3 = unlikely to collect)

Procedure	Initial Evaluations	Ongoing Data Collection	Reevaluations	Dismissal Evaluations
Interview(s)	1	1	1	1
Hearing Screening	1	3; unless the client identifies symptoms	2; depending on length of time since last screening	3
Oral Peripheral Examination	1	3	2	3
Standardized Test(s)	1	3	1	2; initial tests may be readministered for comparison
Observation	1	1	1	1
Structured Interaction(s)	1	1; therapy task is a form of structured interaction	2	3
Dynamic Assessment	1	3	1	3

Why Chart

Table 24–18. Chart Explaining Behaviors a Clinician Might Exhibit in an Assessment and Possible Reasoning Behind These Behaviors

What Was Asked/Done	Why It Was Asked/Done and Possible Reasoning
Ask for parent to sign a consent form.	Legal requirement.
Describe the test or procedure in the report (not just give the name of test).	All readers will understand what was done and what the results mean.
Ask why the client came today (even a child).	Understanding of client's knowledge and what they wish to know.
Fill out the test form completely.	Partial form leads to inaccuracies.
Screen hearing even when no hearing loss is reported.	Client or family may not be aware of the loss. Hearing affects all other communication modalities.
Gather baseline information.	Necessary for comparison purposes and important in billing.
Make referrals.	Communication is just one aspect of the entire person's needs.
Always engage in or observe actual conversation.	Fragmentation of communication into its parts may not accurately reflect the whole.
Proofed for content, spelling, and grammar in every written document.	Accuracy of transmitting information.
Included the highest degree obtained and "CCC-Speech" with the signature on the report.	Providing credentials.

When Chart

Table 24–19. Chart Identifying How You Would Divide Your Time (in 15-min Time Blocks) in an Initial Assessment. Note the Procedure or Tasks of Focus for Each Time Block

Time	Procedure
0–15 min	Opening procedures: introduction, signing permission forms, interview with parents, and description of what assessment will contain. Justification = check accuracy of information, permission must be obtained before anything further can be done, reason for coming and history needed, and information on the process also needed.
16–30 min	Hearing screening; oral peripheral examination. Justification = these assess the integrity of systems used in speech and hearing that could reflect underlying causes; deficits in these could lead to modification in the rest of the assessment.
31–45 min	Standardized articulation test; dynamic assessment articulation (stimulability).
46–60 min	Standardized broad-based language test (expressive and receptive components).
61–75 min	Structured activities of a variety of communication tasks including talking about a book, teaching the clinician how to play a game, and/or informal conversation about school or favorite TV program. Observation of interaction with parent or other family member.
76–90 min	Dynamic assessment and baseline measures of recommended goals.
91–105 min	Scoring tests; discussion with supervisor.
116–120 min	Closing procedure: debrief with parents including any final questions, clarifying results, and recommendations. Justification = family needs to go home with their initial question addressed and an idea of what is next.

Where Chart

Table 24–20. Chart Identifying One or More Places Where an Assessment Would Be Conducted Given a Specific Client Description

Description of Client	Education: Early Intervention, Preschool, K–12, or Colleges/ Universities	Health Care: Nonresidential, Residential, or Hospital	Private Practice: Single Person, Small Practice, or Large Practice
Paul Golden, a 67-year-old male Vietnam veteran, is being evaluated for language abilities following a stroke with an onset of 1 day.		Hospital; VA hospital	
Candy Griffen, a 7-year-old female, is being assessed by an outside agency in order to provide information for a due process hearing from the school.	University clinic	Hospital outpatient services	Private practice
Eddie Worth, a 2;4-year-old male, is being referred for suspected autism.	Early intervention; university clinic	Hospital outpatient	Private practice
Holly Fant, a 20-year-old female with a significant cognitive delay and extended school services, is being reevaluated to update goals and objectives	K–12 school		
Kim Lou, a 30-year-old male physician, is seeking assessment of his articulation to improve his communication skills with clients (note this is not a disorder but a choice to obtain modification of a difference)		Hospital outpatient	Private practice

How Charts (1–10)

Chart 1: Speech sound disorder example (A. G. Bradshaw, personal communication, August 31, 2017). Modifications to include citations were added.

Table 24–21. Speech Sound Disorder Example (A. G. Bradshaw, Personal Communication, August 31, 2017). Modifications to Include Citations Were Added.

Questions to Consider	Answer
Please summarize the intake information from this client (you can make up the specifics of the case you will explore).	10-year-old male. Trouble with /r/ words.
What diagnostic questions are you planning to address?	Is this an articulation error, phonological process error, or motor speech error? Are both vowel and consonant sounds in error? What is the severity level (mild, moderate, or severe)? What is the best therapy approach to recommend?
What are three case-specific questions you will ask in the interview?	When did you first notice the problem? What are some /r/ words he struggles with? Does this affect his overall communication at home and school?
What standardized test(s) do you plan to administer? Why these?	The CAAP-2 (Secord & Donohue, 2013) because it tests both articulation and phonology and is age appropriate. Language and hearing screenings as both are associated with speech sound disorders.
Describe the informal assessment activities you are planning.	Observation and a speech sample. I would ask him to read a portion of an age-appropriate book. Stimulability testing on all errored sounds.
What three specific characteristics do you plan to make note of in an observation time?	What /r/ sounds are affected: initial, medial, or final? Are there other articulation errors or processes present? What is his overall speech intelligibility?
How will you determine recommendations for therapy?	If he scored more than 2 standard deviations below the mean on the test, he would qualify for services. His stimulability score will help determine sounds to target first in treatment. Severity level may impact dosage recommended.
What might be +/− prognostic factors you are going to consider?	Oral peripheral results, stimulability, and hearing results.
How do you plan to get ready to perform this diagnostic (day before, day of, and day following the diagnostic)?	Day before: practice giving the test, organize materials, and review file. Day of: give the tests, interview, observation, and analyze results. Day following: write report and complete billing.

Chart 2: Voice disorder example (A. D. Frady, personal communication, September 20, 2017). Modifications to include citations were added.

Table 24–22. Voice Disorder Example (A. D. Frady, Personal Communication, September 20, 2017). Modifications to Include Citations Were Added.

Questions to Consider	Answer
Please summarize the intake information from this client (you can make up the specifics of the case you will explore).	The client is a 30-year-old, who works as a middle school music teacher and teaches piano and private singing lessons as a side job. Per patient report, she drinks a lot of caffeine (at least four cups per day). She reports rough and breathy voicing as well as pitch breaks. and complains of a sore throat.
What diagnostic questions are you planning to address?	What does the oral-mechanism exam reveal? Are there any noted/apparent abnormalities? Is there symmetry? How is the speed, strength, and range of motion of oral structures? Is there adequate respiration for speech? What is maximum phonation time? What is the s/z ratio? What are the audio-perceptual features? Is there any roughness, breathiness, and/or strain? How is the resonance? How is the client's pitch and loudness? Are there any other abnormalities such as diplophonia, tremor, vocal fry, aphonia, and so forth?
What are three case-specific questions you will ask in the interview?	How does the patient perceive her current voice? Has there been any recent sickness, upper respiratory infections, and so forth to cause a change in voice? Does the patient notice if her symptoms are more severe according to the time of day (e.g., in the morning or after work)?
What standardized test(s) do you plan to administer? Why these?	1) Consensus Auditory-Perceptual Evaluation of Voice (ASHA, 2006): provides perceptual information concerning voice and resonance; may illuminate any additional problems if they are present. 2) Endoscopy: provides confirmation of any structure abnormalities by allowing the clinician to see the anatomy of the vocal folds. 3) CSL (Computerized Speech Lab): provides objective measurements of loudness, pitch, rate, jitter, shimmer, and so forth.

continues

Table 24–22. (*continued*)

Questions to Consider	Answer
Describe the informal assessment activities you are planning.	1) Voice Handicap Index (Jacobson et al., 1997): allows the clinician to understand how the client feels her voice deficits are impacting her overall voice quality and daily life. 2) Observation: provides a subjective analysis of the client's vocal attributes. 3) Interview: provides valuable information as to patient history, how the voice deficits are impacting the client's life, and what the client may want to accomplish through assessment and treatment. 4) Perceptual Tasks: Assess rate, loudness, and pitch to provide observational analysis of voice characteristics. This can be assessed through speaking tasks, s/z ratio, and maximum phonation.
What three specific characteristics do you plan to make note of in an observation time?	Voice quality (roughness, breathiness, etc.), pitch, loudness, rate, and phonation. Is the patient self-conscious of her voice?
How will you determine recommendations for therapy?	Based on objective imaging finding from endoscopy, the clinician will be able to visualize any abnormalities on vocal folds. If any abnormality of the vocal folds is noted, the clinician must refer to an ENT, as SLPs cannot diagnose medically related vocal disorders (vocal nodules, vocal cysts, lesions, etc.). The client is motivated to resume prior level of vocal function and is willing to comply to vocal hygiene plan (e.g., dietary modifications, increased water intake, vocal rest).
What might be +/−prognostic factors you are going to consider?	Client is motivated. Client has prior singing/voice experience. Client understands voicing and respiration coordination. Client's occupation relies on voicing abilities. Noisy work environment with constant vocal demands is a negative factor.
How do you plan to get ready to perform this diagnostic (day before, day of, and day following the diagnostic)?	Day before: have proper equipment ready (endoscopy equipment, CSL lab, etc.). Day of: describe what imaging equipment shows. Discuss any abnormalities and what the next steps are, including a referral if necessary. Day following: make referral calls, if necessary. Have evaluation written up to give to client. Make a follow-up phone call or appointment to discuss evaluation and treatment goals as well as motivation to comply with vocal hygiene plan.

Chart 3: Fluency disorder example (E. E. Lait, personal communication, January 9, 2018). Modifications to include citations were added.

Table 24–23. Fluency Disorder Example (E. E. Lait, Personal Communication, January 9, 2018). Modifications to Include Citations Were Added.

Questions to Consider	Answer
Please summarize the intake information from this client (you can make up the specifics of the case you will explore).	Mike is an intelligent and thoughtful 9-year-old boy whose family has recently moved to the area. He has just transferred to your school and has been referred to you. At his previous school, Mike received speech therapy targeting his stutter. His mother reportedly stuttered as a child but spontaneously recovered in high school. His mother also stated that she is concerned about Mike making friends at his new school due to his insecurities about his stutter. It was reported that Mike had pressure equalization (P.E.) tubes placed in his ears at age 2, but other than that, medical history is unremarkable.
What diagnostic questions are you planning to address?	• Are there any secondary behaviors, such as associated motor behaviors or groping, occurring alongside the stutter? • What is the severity and type of the stutter (e.g., prolongations, part-word repetitions, etc.)? • Do the frequency and types of disfluencies change depending on the setting, situation, and conversational partner(s)? • Are there any negative emotions or avoidance behaviors present that are associated with the disfluencies?
What are three case-specific questions you will ask in the interview?	• When was the initial onset of the stutter? • Was the onset of the stutter connected to an important event in Mike's life (e.g., death in the family)? • Mike has already been receiving intervention services. Have these services been effective? Was there a strategy or type of treatment in particular that seemed to work best for Mike?
What standardized test(s) do you plan to administer? Why these?	• Stuttering Severity Instrument for Adults and Children, Fourth Edition (Riley, 2009): This assessment evaluates frequency of disfluencies (percent disfluency rate), duration of the stuttering events, physical concomitants present, and naturalness of speech.

continues

Table 24–23. (*continued*)

Questions to Consider	Answer
	• Behavior Assessment Battery for School-Age Children Who Stutter (Brutten & Vanryckeghem, 2006): This assessment identifies any emotions and attitudes that the child has associated with the stutter, as well as identifying any coping behaviors that child has developed to deal with his/her stutter. • Screen for speech/language/hearing impairments. • Oral peripheral exam.
Describe the informal assessment activities you are planning.	• Record a conversational speech sample of a length of approximately 30 min. • Record a sample of the child reading age-appropriate material. • Observe Mike in a variety of settings (e.g., classroom, recess, cafeteria). • Send questionnaire home to his parent/guardian to obtain more information about disfluency patterns. • Informal interview/chat with his teacher. Is his stutter interfering with his ability to participate academically?
What three specific characteristics do you plan to make note of in an observation time?	During my observation time, I will make note of the following: ◦ Islands of fluency/instances where the stutter disappears. ◦ Variability of disfluencies depending on the setting and situation. ◦ Does Mike exhibit any avoidance behaviors (e.g., talking around certain words to avoid a stutter)? ◦ Types of disfluencies present. ◦ Abnormal rate of speech.
How will you determine recommendations for therapy?	• When deciding therapy and intervention strategies, I would recommend a group setting for Mike. This would allow him to meet other children who can relate to him and create opportunities for him to make friends, since he is a new transfer and may feel additional social anxiety due to his stutter.
What might be +/− prognostic factors you are going to consider?	Some positive prognostic factors include the fact that Mike has previously received services, seems motivated to participate, and has a family history of spontaneous recovery. Negative prognostic factors include the frequency and severity of stuttering as well as the presence of concomitant motor behaviors such as groping and twitching.

continues

Table 24–23. (continued)

Questions to Consider	Answer
How do you plan to get ready to perform this diagnostic (day before, day of, and day following the diagnostic)?	Day before: review the standardized assessment materials to familiarize myself with the evaluation procedures. I would ensure that all paperwork has been appropriately processed so that I have permission from his parent/guardian to test. Day of: take a few minutes before beginning the assessment procedures to establish rapport with Mike and settle any anxieties he may feel, in order to make sure that the assessment results show the best picture of his capabilities. Day following: draft an IEP and begin making necessary scheduling arrangements to place Mike on my caseload as well as notify the parents of the results.

Chart 4: Language/literacy disorder in children/adolescents example (A. N. Manz, personal communication, September 7, 2017). Modifications to include citations were added.

Table 24–24. Language/Literacy Disorder in Children/Adolescents Example (A. N. Manz, Personal Communication, September 7, 2017). Modifications to Include Citations Were Added.

Questions to Consider	Answer
Please summarize the intake information from this client (you can make up the specifics of the case you will explore).	The client, Kelsey, is a 7-year; 4-month-old female whose first language is English. She was referred to the school SLP by her first grade teacher. Her teacher reports that Kelsey often "stares blankly" when asked a direct question and gives unrelated answers or declines answering. The teacher also stated that Kelsey has difficulty following whole-class directions and has trouble remembering vocabulary from the content taught in class from one day to the next. The short questionnaire sent home to Kelsey's parents revealed that she attended private preschool for 2 years because they "thought she just wasn't quite ready for kindergarten." Kelsey passed her hearing screening at the beginning of the year. Both her teacher and her parents report that Kelsey is a happy, curious girl. Her teacher reports that she is very timid around her peers except for two close friends in class.

continues

Table 24–24. (continued)

Questions to Consider	Answer
What diagnostic questions are you planning to address?	Does Kelsey present with a receptive language disorder, expressive language disorder, both, or neither? How are her language difficulties affecting her academically? What differences, if any, can be seen in Kelsey's language skills across settings or conversational partners? How is Kelsey's comprehension when presented with material she is already familiar with versus new material?
What are three case-specific questions you will ask in the interview?	Does Kelsey have a history of ear infections? Is there a family history of language problems? Describe a couple situations in daily life where you feel like communication often breaks down with Kelsey (e.g., giving directions, family dinner conversation, talking about school).
What standardized test(s) do you plan to administer? Why these?	I would do a comprehensive language tests such as the CELF-5 (Wiig, Semel, & Second, 2013) or TOLD-P:4 (Newcomer & Hammill, 2008) in order to get an overall picture of Kelsey's receptive and expressive language strengths and needs. I would also give the EOWPVT-4 and ROWPVT-4 (Brownell, 2012) since the teacher specifically indicated difficulty with vocabulary. Her performance on the ROW-PVT can also help determine whether her difficulty with receptive language tasks (answering questions, following directions) stems from deficits in receptive semantics or if complexity of syntax is more of an issue. If receptive semantics is within normal limits (WNL), criterion-referenced measures of syntax could be administered to determine specific areas of need.
Describe the informal assessment activities you are planning.	Simple board game (e.g., Trouble, Connect 4); generate conversation throughout. Open-ended activity such as coloring/drawing; generate conversation throughout.
What three specific characteristics do you plan to make note of in an observation time?	Kelsey's use of more complex syntax. Kelsey's understanding of more complex/less common syntax (e.g., passive instead of active voice). Kelsey's ability to follow one-, two-, and three-step directions during informal activities.
How will you determine recommendations for therapy?	In many school districts, eligibility for speech-language services are determined by standard scores. If Kelsey is within the range of eligibility based on standard measures and I saw evidence of deficits in interview, observation, and informal assessment, I would likely

continues

Table 24–24. (continued)

Questions to Consider	Answer
	recommend therapy. Goals would be determined by areas of need evidenced by the aforementioned assessment measures, while taking into account those tasks that would most benefit Kelsey academically.
What might be +/– prognostic factors you are going to consider?	I would look at family history of language disorders, severity of Kelsey's impairment according to standardized and informal assessment measures, and Kelsey's performance on dynamic assessment measures. Kelsey's ability to use supports and strategies independently or with minimal cueing would be a positive prognostic indicator.
How do you plan to get ready to perform this diagnostic (day before, day of, and day following the diagnostic)?	Day before: make sure I have all the student information I need, ensure I have any parent/teacher questionnaires returned from the parent/teacher (and if not, I would contact them), and ensure I have all the components of the standardized tests I plan to give as well as materials ready for informal assessment. If I am not familiar or comfortable with a certain measure, I would take time to review the manual, materials, and protocols. I would also ensure I have permission to record if I am planning to do so.
	Day of: there should not be much to do to prepare because I organized everything yesterday. If working in a school setting, I would remind the teacher of the time the student would be pulled for testing and make sure the student is not absent that day.
	Day following: check to make sure I am not missing any key pieces of information needed to determine treatment recommendations, and, if I am missing information, I would try to obtain it prior to writing the assessment report.

Chart 5: Language disorder in adults example (D. E. Carter, personal communication, December 10, 2017). Modifications to include citations were added.

Table 24–25. Language Disorder in Adults Example (D. E. Carter, Personal Communication, December 10, 2017). Modifications to Include Citations Were Added.

Questions to Consider	Answer
Please summarize the intake information from this client (you can make up the specifics of the case you will explore).	The client is a 61-year-old male who came into the outpatient clinic complaining of difficulties with his speech. His wife mentioned that he had a stroke 6 months ago caused by occlusion to the middle cerebral artery of the inferior posterior frontal lobe of the left hemisphere. He is married and has two children who are in college. The wife is concerned about his speaking skills which sound telegraphic. His speaking is effortful and labored and composed of many misarticulations.
What diagnostic questions are you planning to address?	What type of aphasia does this client present with? What goals/objectives does the client personally want to achieve? What treatment plan/methods will be most beneficial for this client?
What are three case-specific questions you will ask in the interview?	When did the stroke occur? How much spontaneous recovery has occurred since the stroke happened? What would you say are your strengths in communication?
What standardized test(s) do you plan to administer? Why these?	The Aphasia Diagnostic Profile (ADP) (Helm-Estabrooks, 1992) will be administered to assess communication and language impairment through nine different subtests. This test is a standardized test that allows comparison of scores to norms and provides guidance for future therapy based on weaknesses identified in the assessment. The Stroke and Aphasia Quality of Life Scale-39 (SAQOL-39) (Hilari & Byng, 2003) will be administered to assess the patient's self-reports of what is important in terms of his recovery and to help guide therapy to meet his goals and improve his quality of life post stroke. The American Speech-Language-Hearing Association's Functional Assessment of Communication Skills for Adults (ASHA FACS) (Frattali, Thompson, Holland, Wohl, & Ferketic, 1995) will be administered to further assess the patient's functional communication abilities.

continues

Table 24–25. *(continued)*

Questions to Consider	Answer
Describe the informal assessment activities you are planning.	A patient interview will be conducted to obtain pertinent information regarding medical history, case history, concerns that lead to the request for the assessment, and if a communication disorder is evident. This interview will serve as a conversational speech sample. An oral facial exam will also be conducted to inspect function and structure of the articulators. Voice quality will be noted along with any apparent difficulties with hearing.
What three specific characteristics do you plan to make note of in an observation time?	1) Confrontation naming ability 2) Repetition skills 3) Auditory comprehension 4) Reading skills 5) Writing skills
How will you determine recommendations for therapy?	Based on the scores from the informal and formal language measures, the recommendation for beginning therapy will be determined. If therapy is indicated, then goals and objectives will be recommended for targets based off of the information gathered in the assessment.
What might be +/– prognostic factors you are going to consider?	The client's motivation, enthusiasm, and thoughts on improving will all be prognostic factors along with the client's support system.
How do you plan to get ready to perform this diagnostic (day before, day of, and day following the diagnostic)?	The day before, I will make sure to go over the tests to familiarize myself with them. I will ensure that all paperwork is ready to test the client. The day of will consist of making copies of necessary materials and gathering items for the assessment and writing the report after the assessment. The day after will be comprised of making edits to the report that was written the previous day and billing, along with following up by calling the spouse or family.

Chart 6: Cognitive disorder example (T. D. McKinney, personal communication, October 23, 2017). Modifications to include citations were added.

Table 24–26. Cognitive Disorder Example (T. D. McKinney, Personal Communication, October 23, 2017). Modifications to Include Citations Were Added.

Questions to Consider	Answer
Please summarize the intake information from this client (you can make up the specifics of the case you will explore).	Client is a 27-year-old female with a traumatic brain injury (TBI) following a motor vehicle accident. She was hospitalized at WakeMed hospital for 3 months and received intensive inpatient rehabilitation while there. The client now lives at home with her mother and younger sister. Her family reported that the client is easily distracted both in conversation and while reading. The client has difficulty recalling information shortly after it is delivered. She also has poor orientation skills.
What diagnostic questions are you planning to address?	How long ago did your motor vehicle accident occur? Have you noticed any word-finding issues? Can you tell me about your experience with speech therapy in the past? What kind of things did you work on? Can you independently complete activities of daily living (ADLs)?
What are three case-specific questions you will ask in the interview?	How often to do notice your brain injury negatively effecting your everyday life? What are some examples of these situations? What is your number one goal if therapy is needed?
What standardized test(s) do you plan to administer? Why these?	I plan to administer the Scales of Cognitive Ability for Traumatic Brain Injury (SCATBI; Adamovich & Henderson, 1992) and portions of the Ross Information Processing Assessment, Second Edition (RIPA-2; Ross-Swain, 1996) that target memory. The SCATBI covers the areas of perception/discrimination, orientation, organization, recall, and reasoning. I would administer this assessment because it targets not only the areas mentioned by the client and family, but also other areas that are commonly impaired in persons with TBIs. I would administer the memory portions of the RIPA-2 to further assess her recall and memory skills since this was a concern from the beginning.
Describe the informal assessment activities you are planning.	I would administer the Boston Naming Test (Kaplan, Goodglass & Weintraub, 1983) if the patient complained of word-finding issues. Although this is not a standardized test, it would give me the information needed to know if word-finding should be targeted in

continues

Table 24–26. *(continued)*

Questions to Consider	Answer
	therapy. I would also engage the client in conversation to observe her pragmatic skills including the use of gestures, eye contact, topic maintenance, facial expressions, and understanding of facial expressions and gestures. Lastly, I would give her a reading passage to read aloud to observe attentional deficits mentioned by the client and family.
What three specific characteristics do you plan to make note of in an observation time?	What are some examples of the client's poor recall skills? What kinds of questions are you asking? Do you notice a certain time of day or environment that tends to cause more difficulty for the client? What are some examples of the client's poor orientation skills?
How will you determine recommendations for therapy?	I will determine recommendations for therapy based on the strengths and weaknesses found from the formal and informal assessments as well as the observation. Personal goals from the client will also be highly considered. For example, if the client's main goal is to return to school for cosmetology, then the therapy activities can be centered around that goal by addressing attention, recall, and orientation in a functional manner.
What might be +/− prognostic factors you are going to consider?	Positive prognostic factors include motivation and supportive family system. Negative prognostic factors would be the length of time it has been since the accident occurred.
How do you plan to get ready to perform this diagnostic (day before, day of, and day following the diagnostic)?	Day before: I will do a thorough chart review of the client. I will also look over the tests I am going to give to make sure I know how to properly give the assessments. Day of: I will have everything set up before the client arrives and have backup tasks and assessments in case the client does not present the way I anticipated. Day following: I will look over the assessment scores, recall the information from the informal assessment and observation, research, and conclude if therapy is warranted, the frequency of therapy, and the goals of therapy.

Chart 7: Social communication disorder example (N. T. Greenway, personal communication, February 18, 2018). Modifications to include citations were added.

Table 24–27. Social Communication Disorder Example (N. T. Greenway, Personal Communication, February 18, 2018). Modifications to Include Citations Were Added.

Questions to Consider	Answer
Please summarize the intake information from this client (you can make up the specifics of the case you will explore).	The client moved to a new school district at the beginning of the previous school year. He was receiving therapy at his previous school and has an active IEP targeting receptive and expressive language skills. His second grade teacher has requested that he be evaluated for a possible social communication disorder. His teacher noted that he seems to have difficulty interacting with other classmates appropriately and expresses his frustration in a negative way, often screaming at his peers and having difficulty taking the perspective of others when he is upset. No case history or other information was transferred with the student to the new school, just the objectives his previous SLP was targeting in therapy.
What diagnostic questions are you planning to address?	– How is this possible social communication disorder affecting the student in the classroom? – Is the student aware of his social communication difficulties or does he feel that there is no present problem? – If the student is aware of his difficulties, what does he feel he could improve on in order to communicate with his classmates more effectively? – What do I, as the SLP, notice during the diagnostic session that are potential red flags for a social communication disorder?
What are three case-specific questions you will ask in the interview?	– Do you feel that you communicate your emotions in a way that is appropriate? – How do you know that someone is happy? How do you know that someone is upset? – What are some ways we can gain control of our emotions when we are upset?
What standardized test(s) do you plan to administer? Why these?	Since the student came with goals written by a previous speech therapist, I would reevaluate his speech and language in order to update his goals and to see if either

continues

Table 24–27. *(continued)*

Questions to Consider	Answer
	of those disorders could be contributing to his possible social communication disorder. I would evaluate his speech using the Goldman-Fristoe Test of Articulation, Third Edition (GFTA-3; Goldman & Fristoe, 2015). This is a quick test that rules out articulation disorders for any school-aged client. I would assess his language skills using the Clinical Evaluation of Language Fundamentals, Fifth Edition (CELF-5; Wiig, Semel, & Secord, 2013). This assessment measures a variety of topics that I think are beneficial in ruling out an expressive or receptive language delay. The CELF-5 also contains a pragmatics profile, which is a parent/teacher questionnaire that I believe would be valuable to obtain. Lastly, I would administer the Test of Pragmatic Language-2 (TOPL-2) (Phelps-Terasaki & Phelps-Gunn, 2007). This assessment measure is mostly comprised of questions that deal with polite conduct. If I felt it was necessary, I would consider also administering the Social Emotional Evaluation (SEE) (Wiig, 2008), which involves recalling facial expressions and identifying emotions.
Describe the informal assessment activities you are planning.	I would begin informally assessing the student by viewing him interacting with peers in a variety of environments, both structured and unstructured. I might choose to watch him interact in the classroom, on the playground, at lunch, and during a special class where there might be more communication with peers, such as art or P.E. I would also interview his parents and teachers with regards to his social cognition and behaviors to gain their perspective on his strengths and needs. I might provide the parents or teachers with the Children's Communication Checklist-2 (CCC-2)(Bishop, 2006), which addresses pragmatic aspects of communication as well as other related behaviors. Next, I would have a structured interaction with the student where I would ask him questions and allow him to ask me questions, focusing on gauging his awareness of his social communication difficulties. I would do a problem solving task and an emotion recognition task with him to identify any problems in those areas, as those are some of the fundamental skills for social competence.

continues

Table 24–27. *(continued)*

Questions to Consider	Answer
What five specific characteristics do you plan to make note of in an observation time?	– His ability to gauge peers' feelings during structured and unstructured interactions. – How he seems to initiate interaction with peers. – His awareness of his expression of emotions when upset. – How he expresses his frustration with peers. – His skills in the structured therapy tasks (problem solving and social recognition) and his willingness to comply with therapeutic activities.
How will you determine recommendations for therapy?	I will use the results from the standardized assessment measures as well as the informal assessments. I will take into consideration the parent and teacher interviews, how he interacted with peers, and what I noticed during structured therapy activities. Since social communication disorders present in a variety of characteristics and severities, I will need to incorporate all information from the diagnostic sessions in order to provide a strong case if I feel social communication therapy is warranted for this student.
What might be +/– prognostic factors you are going to consider?	A positive prognostic factor would be if he uses age-appropriate greetings and farewells when conversing with classmates and adults, myself included. I would also consider his ability to engage in conversation with peers and adults, his ability to repair breakdowns in conversation, and his skills of understanding both verbal and nonverbal signals from others. Lastly, I would take into consideration his understanding of figurative language and ability to infer.
How do you plan to get ready to perform this diagnostic (day before, day of, and day following the diagnostic)?	Day before: try to have the parent and teacher interviews completed. This would give me a good understanding of the student before beginning the diagnostic session. Day of: gather my diagnostic materials and determine with his teacher the best time to do observations. Day following: provide diagnostic results and recommendations to his parents and his teachers.

Chart 8: Communication modality disorder example (K. L. McDonald-Coxen, personal communication, February 18, 2018). Modifications to include citations were added.

Table 24–28. Communication Modality Disorder Example (K. L. McDonald-Coxen, Personal Communication, February 18, 2018). Modifications to Include Citations Were Added.

Questions to Consider	Answer
Please summarize the intake information from this client (you can make up the specifics of the case you will explore).	This client is a child of 5 years who has cerebral palsy and has a diagnosis of severe dysarthria; some apraxic-like groping is present. Functionally, the child has age-appropriate receptive language and minimal expressive language with average pragmatic skills. The child is able to complete most age-appropriate gross motor movements independently, but has difficulty with fine motor skills due to incoordination and some weakness. This client attends school in a regular classroom and has an aid to assist. The child's parents aren't happy with the progress their child has made despite speech therapy since the age of 3 and want to try a speech generation device.
What diagnostic questions are you planning to address?	I will determine the impact of dysarthria and apraxia on the child speech as well as expressive and receptive language.
	I will assess the viability of the child using AAC to improve participation in class.
What are three case-specific questions you will ask in the interview?	I will ask the parents to describe the child's birth and onset of symptoms.
	I will ask what the family's long-term goal is for their child with regard to communication.
	I will ask what strategies are in place in the classroom thus far to assist with communication success.
What standardized test(s) do you plan to administer? Why these?	I plan to give the Preschool Language Scales, Fifth Edition (Zimmerman, Steiner, & Pond, 2011) to determine the child's receptive and expressive language skills.

continues

Table 24–28. *(continued)*

Questions to Consider	Answer
Describe the informal assessment activities you are planning.	I will set up a play area with some enticing age-appropriate toys such as bubbles and blocks. Ideally, the child will be able to play with a sibling or family member so I can observe the child in a more relaxed setting and try to gather a good conversational sample.
	I will conduct an oral mechanism exam and interview the parents or guardians about their child's communicative strengths and weaknesses. If possible, I will have some trial AAC devices for the child to use, since that is something the parent's expressed they want to try.
What three specific characteristics do you plan to make note of in an observation time?	I plan to take note of the severity of the dysarthria in speech, intelligibility, use of nonverbal gestures and expressions, and general play skills.
How will you determine recommendations for therapy?	I will base my recommendations for therapy on the results of the standardized assessments, dynamic measures, observation, and the needs of the parents and child. I will try to balance what makes sense for this family with school-related needs.
What might be +/– prognostic factors you are going to consider?	I will consider family investment in therapy, financial considerations (as AAC can be very expensive), and the support from the school. It will be important to have teacher and staff buy into these considerations help the child communicate successfully with AAC.
How do you plan to get ready to perform this diagnostic (day before, day of, and day following the diagnostic)?	Day before: make sure I am familiar with the specifics of the standardized protocols I will use and collect forms such as parent interview questions and patient history.
	Day of: set out play items and set up the room where the evaluation will take place as well as gather appropriate intake forms I've prepared the day before.
	Day following: compile results into a formal evaluation and contact the parents/caregivers for a follow-up session where I will share my recommendations. If an electronic AAC device or application is seen as a good fit, I will begin the paperwork depending on the device the family chooses to hopefully obtain funding.

Chart 9: Audiology disorder example (M. E. Momphard, personal communication, December 6, 2017). Modifications to include citations were added.

Table 24–29. Audiology Disorder Example (M. E. Momphard, Personal Communication, December 6, 2017). Modifications to Include Citations Were Added.

Audiology

Questions to Consider	Answer
Please summarize the intake information from this client (you can make up the specifics of the case you will explore).	Mr. Jones is a 59-year-old male who is complaining of difficulty hearing. He reported that his right ear is his "good ear." He first noticed the hearing loss around five years ago, and it has progressively worsened. As a young child, Mr. Jones had two ear infections. He has never had a serious head injury or ear surgery. Mr. Jones first consulted his primary care physician about his difficulty hearing 2 weeks ago; he was given a referral to an audiologist for a complete hearing assessment. Mr. Jones does not have a family history of hearing loss. He also complains of hearing ringing in his ears when no noise is present, but does not report feelings of dizziness. He does not have a history of serious illnesses, and is not currently taking any medications. Mr. Jones is presently employed. He works in construction as a foreman. He reports difficulty understanding speech both on the job and at home.
What diagnostic questions are you planning to address?	The type and severity of the hearing loss as well as the underlying cause.
What are three case-specific questions you will ask in the interview?	– Does he wear hearing protection on the job? How often and what type? – What sort of environments does Mr. Jones have difficulty discriminating speech in? Quiet with background noise, and/or in loud environments? Does he have difficulty hearing pure tones? – Does he feel that the reported hearing loss has a negative impact on his life? In what way (with family, with acquaintances, on the job)?

continues

Table 24–29. (continued)

Questions to Consider	Answer
What standardized test(s) do you plan to administer? Why these?	– Audiogram (to determine type and severity of hearing loss) – Tympanometry (to aid in narrowing down the possible causes of hearing loss) – Speech discrimination test (to determine how well Mr. Jones is hearing spoken language)
What three specific characteristics do you plan to make note of in an observation time?	– Apparent ease of conversation with familiar conversational partner. – Apparent ease of conversation with unfamiliar conversational partner. – Willingness to contribute to conversation.
How will you determine recommendations for therapy?	If Mr. Jones has poor word recognition (relative to his performance on the audiogram) or experiences increase difficulty listening in noisy environments, I would recommend auditory therapy.
What might be +/– prognostic factors you are going to consider?	– Desire to improve communication. (+) – Willingness to wear hearing aids. (+) – Willingness to wear hearing protection at work. (+) – Other comorbid conditions. (–)
How do you plan to get ready to perform this diagnostic (day before, day of, and day following the diagnostic)?	Day before: – Review the intake questionnaire and compile a list of questions to ask Mr. Jones in the interview. – Prepare the equipment and materials needed to perform the assessments. Day of: – Complete an interview with the client. – Perform the tests. – Score the tests. Day following: – Analyze and write the report. – Bill insurance.

Chart 10: Swallowing disorder example (R. A. Cox, personal communication, October 23, 2017). Modifications to include citations were added.

Table 24–30. Swallowing Disorder Example (R. A. Cox, Personal Communication, October 23, 2017). Modifications to Include Citations Were Added.

Questions to Consider	Answer
Please summarize the intake information from this client (you can make up the specifics of the case you will explore).	Amy is a 52-year-old female who is happily married with two children. On Mondays and Wednesdays, she serves at a local church where she is the secretary. For the past 6 months, she has noticed that her body is changing. Both her and her family have noticed the following: loss of coordination; weak muscles; vocal pitch changes; slurred speech; muscle cramping; periods of uncontrollable laughing and crying; breathing difficulties; and trouble walking long distances. Amy's physician referred her to a neurologist where she received the diagnosis of amyotrophic lateral sclerosis (ALS). After receiving the diagnosis, a couple weeks later she began noticing difficulties swallowing. Not only does she have difficulties eating and drinking, but sometimes, especially late at night, she has trouble swallowing her own saliva. In addition, her husband reported that she consistently drools. Her neurologist referred her to see a SLP to have a swallowing evaluation. Two weeks before her speech therapy appointment, Amy was diagnosed with pneumonia and is currently taking antibiotics.
What diagnostic questions are you planning to address?	Are there atypical parameters of structures and functions affecting the swallow mechanism? Is the ALS affecting her overall swallowing mechanism? If so, how? What are the effects of the swallowing impairment on the individual's activities and participation? Are there any contextual factors that serve as barriers to or facilitators of successful swallowing? Is dysphagia present? What phase of swallowing is being affected? Oral? Pharyngeal? Esophageal? Is penetration or aspiration occurring? Is a diet modification needed? What is the best recommendation for intervention? What is her prognosis for improvement? Should she be referred to any other services or professionals (counseling, OT, etc.)?

continues

Table 24–30. (*continued*)

Questions to Consider	Answer
What are 3 case specific questions you will ask in the interview?	Do you have episodes of coughing when eating/drinking? Do you ever feel as if food/drink "goes down the wrong way"? Do you ever feel as if food gets stuck in your throat?
What standardized test(s) do you plan to administer? Why these?	Instrumental Swallowing Assessments: Videofluoroscopy swallowing study (VFSS), also known as a modified barium swallow study (MBSS). VFSS can be done either independently by a trained SLP or by an SLP in addition with other members of the team. This provides a direct lateral view of the oral, pharyngeal, and upper esophageal function. This allows the bolus to be visualized in real time on an x-ray during the swallow. This allows the SLP to identify whether penetration and/or aspiration occurred as well as view the anatomy and pathophysiology of the swallow function in the various phases. In addition, this assessment provides useful information on the influence of compensatory strategies and diet changes. Amyotrophic Lateral Sclerosis Severity Scale (Hillel et al., 1989): This helps provide an ordinal staging system and a mean of assessment for individuals with ALS. It allows the clinician to look at the symptoms of ALS in four categories, swallowing being one domain. This provides an accurate assessment of the patient's disease status and can be effective in treatment planning and prognosis monitoring. Mann Assessment of Swallowing (Mann, 2002): This provides a number score that is used to represent the severity of dysphagia and aspiration present.
Describe the informal assessment activities are you planning?	Noninstrumental Swallowing Assessments: Interview/case history Oral mechanism examination Review of past medical and clinical records including the potential impact of current medications Assessment of speech and vocal quality at baseline and any changes following bolus or liquid presentations Assessment of Amy's perception of function, severity, overall quality of life, and so forth

continues

Table 24–30. (*continued*)

Questions to Consider	Answer
	Evaluation of the method and rate of bolus presentation and the effects on swallowing
	Observation of secretion management skills (frequency)
	Observation of Amy eating various consistencies
	Observation of any signs/symptoms of penetration and/or aspiration
	Observation of respiratory rate and the respiratory/swallowing pattern
	Cervical auscultation
	Hyoid/laryngeal palpation evaluation of cough strength

What 3 specific characteristics do you plan to make note of in an observation time?	Observation would occur during a meal time, if possible. If not, the clinician will present various bolus and liquid consistencies and observe the client eating. Here are five characteristics that the clinician would plan on observing
	  1) Does the patient cough during or shortly after swallowing?
	  2) Is there speech or vocal quality changes that occur following bolus/liquid presentations?
	  3) What is the preferred method of presentation to the client (self-fed, spoon, cup, examiner-fed, etc.)?
	  4) How is the client's oral preparation? Is there adequate labial seal? Is there evidence of oral control?
	  5) What is the amount of time required to complete the swallow sequence? Is fatigue noted toward the end of the meal or with certain bolus consistencies?

How will you determine recommendations for therapy?	Results of the formal and informal assessment measures. Severity of her ALS score. Patient and family treatment desires. Research peer-reviewed journal articles that discuss this same topic
What might be +/- prognostic factors you are going to consider?	Is the client and her family receptive and open to various bolus and liquid consistencies? Is the client willing to participate in therapy? Is the dysphagia characterized in the oral prep, oral, pharyngeal, or esophageal stage? What is her ALS severity level?

continues

Table 24–30. *(continued)*

Questions to Consider	Answer
How do you plan to get ready to perform this diagnostic (day before, day of, and day following the diagnostic)?	Day before: conduct phone interview with the client to gain basic information. Have the client return case history forms and then review them. Contact the client's neurologist/family doctor to gather more information, if necessary. Contact the local VFSS agency used and schedule a time for the evaluation. Day of: gather and prepare various food consistencies. Gather materials needed for the assessments (pen light, tongue swab, flashlight, etc.). Complete the assessment. Day following: complete the diagnostic report. Make recommendations and treatment goals. Contact the family to schedule a follow-up appointment to discuss the results.

References

Adamovich, B. B., & Henderson, J. (1992). Scales of cognitive ability for traumatic brain injury (SCATBI) [Assessment instrument]. Austin, TX: Pro-Ed.

ASHA. (n.d.). Employment settings for SLPs. Retrieved May 22, 2018, from https://www.asha.org/Students/Employment-Settings-for-SLPs/

ASHA. (2006). Consensus auditory-perceptual evaluation of voice (CAPE-V) [Assessment instrument]. Retrieved from https://www.asha.org/uploadedFiles/members/divs/D3CAPEVprocedures.pdf

Bishop, D. (2006). Children communication checklist -2 (CCC-2). [Assessment instrument]. New York City, N.Y. :Pearson.

Brownell, R. (2012). Receptive and expressive one-word picture vocabulary tests (4th ed.) (ROWPVT-4 and EOWPVT-4) [Assessment instrument]. San Antonio, TX: PsychCorp.

Brutten, G. J., & Vanryckeghem, M. (2006). Behavior assessment battery for school age children who stutter (BAB) [Assessment instrument]. San Diego, CA: Plural Publishing Inc.

Carrow-Wollfork, E. (2011). Oral and written language scales (2nd ed.) (OWLS-II) [Assessment instrument]. San Antonio, TX: PsychCorp.

Carrow-Woolfork, E. (2017). Comprehensive assessment of spoken language (2nd ed.) (CASL-2) [Assessment instrument]. Austin, TX: Pro-Ed.

Dodd, B., Hua, Z., Crosbie, S., Holm, A., & Ozanne, A. (2006). Diagnostic evaluation of articulation and phonology (DEAP) [Assessment instrument]. San Antonio, TX: PsychCorp.

Dunn, L. M., & Dunn, D. M. (2007). Peabody picture vocabulary test (4th ed.) (PPVT-4) [Assessment instrument]. San Antonio, TX: PsychCorp. https://www.asha.org/Students/Employment-Settings-for-SLPs/

Frattali, C. M., Thompson, C. K., Holland, A. L., Wohl, C. B., & Ferketic, M. M. (1995). *The American Speech-Language-Hearing Association Functional Assessment of Communication Skills for Adults (ASHA FACS).* [Assessment instrument]. Rockville, MD: ASHA.

Goldman, R., & Fristoe, M. (2015). Goldman-Fristoe test of articulation (3rd ed.) (GFTA-3) [Assessment instrument]. Austin, TX: Pro-Ed.

Helm-EstaBrooks, N. (1992) Aphasia Diagnostic Profiles (ADP) [Assessment instrument]. Austin, TX: Pro-Ed.

Helm-Estabrooks, N. (2001). Cognitive linguistic quick test-plus (CLQT+) [Assessment instrument]. San Antonio, TX: PsychCorp.

Hilari, K & Byng, S. (2001). Measuring quality of life in people with aphasia: the Stroke Specific Quality of Life Scale. Int J Lang Commun.Disord; 36 Suppl:86-91 [Assessment instrument].

Hillel, A. D., Miller R. M., Yorkston, K., McDonald E., Norris, F. H., & Konikow, N. (1989). Amyotrophic lateral sclerosis severity scale (ALSSS) Neuroepidemiology. 8(3), 142-50 (PubMed Abstracts)[Assessment instrument].

Jacobson, B. H., Johnson, A., Grywalski, C., Silbergleit, A., Jacobson, G., Benninger, M. S., & Newman, C. W. (1997). The voice handicap index (VHI): Development and validation. *American Journal of Speech-Language Pathology*, *6*(3), 66–69.

Kaplan, E., Goodglass, H., & Weintraub, S. (1983). The Boston naming test [Assessment instrument]. Philadelphia, PA: Le & Febiger.

Kertesz, A. (2007). Western aphasia battery-revised (WAB-R) [Assessment instrument]. San Antonio, TX: PsychCorp.

Mann, G. (2002). Mann assessment of swallowing (MASA) [Assessment instrument]. Stamford, CT: Thomson Learning, Inc.

Newcomer, P. L., & Hammill, D. D. (2008). Test of language development-primary (4th ed.) (TOLD-P:4) [Assessment instrument]. Austin, TX: Pro-Ed.

Phelps-Teraski, D. & Phelps-Gunn, T. (2007). Test of pragmatic language (2nd ed.) (TOPL-2) [Assessment instrument]. Novato, CA: Academic Therapy Publications.

Riley, G. (2009). The stuttering severity instrument for adults and children (4th ed.) (SSI-4) [Assessment instrument]. Austin, TX: Pro-Ed.

Ross-Swain, D. (1996). Ross information processing assessment (2nd ed.) (RIPA-2) [Assessment instrument]. Austin, TX: Pro-Ed.

Secord, W., & Donohue, J. (2013). Clinical assessment of articulation and phonological (2nd ed.) (CAAP-2) [Assessment instrument]. Austin, TX: Pro-Ed.

Wiig, E.H. (2008). Social emotional evaluation (SEE) [Assessment Instrument]. Austin, TX. Pro-Ed.

Wiig, E. H., Semel, E., & Second, W. (2013). Clinical evaluation of language fundamentals (5th ed.) (CELF-5) [Assessment instrument]. San Antonio, TX: PsychCorp.

Zimmerman, I. L., Steiner, V. G., & Pond, R. E. (2011). Preschool language scales (5th ed.) (PLS-5). [Assessment instrument]. San Antonio, TX: PyschCorp.

Index

Note: Page numbers in **bold** reference non-text material.

A

AAC. *See* Augmentative and alternative communication
Activities
   for adult language assessment, 201–202
   assessment, 3–4
   for billing, 131–134
   for cognitive assessment, 211–213
   for dynamic assessment, 65–66
   for dysphagia assessment, 181–182
   for fluency assessment, 171–172
   for health insurance, 142–145
   for hearing assessment, 119–123
   for initial interviews, 24–26
   for language/literacy, 192–197
   for modalities, communication, 233–235
   observation, 73–75
   for ongoing assessment, 110–112
   for oral-facial examinations, 36–40
   referral, 13–16
   for report writing, 98–100
   for social communication assessment, 221–225
   for speech sound disorders, 153–156
   for standardized tests/testing, 48–49
   for statistical information, 57–58
   for synthesizing information, 85–86
   for voice assessment, 163–164
Adult language assessment. *See also* Aphasia
   activities for, 201–202
   wrap-ups for, 201–205
Adult language disorders, standardized tests for, 199
Age-equivalent scores, 46
Aided/unaided help, 230
Anatomical structures, **39–40**
Anomia, 198
Antecedent events, 69
Aphasia
   assessment methods for, 199–200
   categorizing, 197–198
      fluent, 198
      nonfluent, 197–198
   characteristics tied with, 198
   defined, 197
   evaluation settings for, 198–199
   reasons for assessing, 198
   timing of assessment for, 198
Appearances, observation as, 69
Apraxia of speech, childhood, diagnosing, 149–150
Articulation errors, defined, 149
Assessment
   activities for, 3–4
   wrap-ups for, 5–7
Assessment Information section, 92–93
Assessments. *See also specific types of assessment*
   places for, 2
   questions for clinicians in, 1–2
   reasons for, 2
   timing of, 2
Assistive technology resource centers (ATRCs), 231
Augmentative and alternative communication (AAC)
   aided vs. unaided help in, 230
   diseases containing component of, 229
   interviews in, 230
   observation for, 231
   questionnaires in, 230
   standardized testing for, 230–231
   structured interactions for, 231
Augmentative and alternative communication (AAC) devices, 230
Augmentative and alternative communication (AAC) evaluations
   reasons for, 231
   timing of, 231
Augmentative and alternative communication (AAC) strategies, 229–231
Authentic assessment, 218

Authentic component, of language/literacy evaluation, 189
Autism spectrum diagnosis, 219

B

Basal items, 45
Baseline assessments, 2
Bedside examinations, 179
　checklist for, 184–186
Behaviors, reporting information on, 69–70
Bilingual clients, 82
Billing, 125
　activities for, 131–134
　form, 127–128, **128**
　HCFA 1500 form, 128, **129–130**
　procedures, reasons for learning, 126–127
　systems of
　　Current Procedural Terminology (CPT) codes, 126
　　Healthcare Common Procedures Coding System (HCPCS) codes, 126
　　International Classification of Diseases, 10th Revision, Clinical Modification (ICD-10 CM), 125–126
　timing of, 127
　　for health insurance, 139–140
　wrap-ups for, 134–135
Bridging questions, 63

C

Calibration
　of audiological equipment, 117
　of instruments, 107
Case histories, 82
　for aphasia assessment, 199
　assessing fluency disorders and, 169
　for dysphagia assessments, 179
　for social communication disorders, 220
　voice assessment and, 160
Ceiling items, 47
Charts, 54–55
　ability to read, 53
Chronological age, determining, 55
Client-appropriate tests, defined, 43
Clinical questions, 1
Clinicians, assessment questions for, 1–2
Closed-head injuries, 207–208
Cluttering, 167, 168
Cochlear implant surgery, 116
Coding modifiers, 126
　G-Codes, 127

Cognitive assessments, 207–208
　activities for, 211–213
　methods of, 209–210
　reasons for, 208
　settings for, 208
　timing of, 208
　wrap-ups for, 213–215
Communication disorders, 2
Computerized Speech Labs, 162
Conductive hearing loss, 116
Confidence intervals, 46
Confirmation-refining function, 70
Consequences, 69
Correct coding initiatives, 139
Correlation, 54
Counts, observation as, 69
Current Procedural Terminology (CPT) codes, 126

D

Data generation, forms of, 107–108
Dementia, defined, 208
Demographic information, 9
Development disabilities (DDs), 207
Diadochokinetic rate (DDK), evaluation of, 34
Diagnostic codes, billing system for, 125–126
Diagnosticians. *See* Clinicians
Disfluencies, 167
Disfluency index, 169–170
Durable medical equipment, coding for, 126
Duration, 106
Dynamic assessments, 2, 61
　activities for, 65–66
　for augmentative and communication evaluations, 231
　defined, 61–62
　focus of, 62–63
　as gage, 62
　of language/literacy, 188
　methodology of, 63
　organized plan for, 63, **64**
　settings for, 63
　test-teach-test form of, 61–62
　timing of, 63
　wrap-ups for, 66–68
Dysarthria, childhood, 149–150
Dysphagia
　assessment activities for, 181–182
　assessment techniques, 179–180
　phases of
　　oral preparatory phase, 177

oral, 177
 pharyngeal, 177
 esophageal, 177
 screening for, 177–178
 settings for screenings of, 178
 timing of screenings for, 18
 wrap-ups for, 182–186

E

Echolalia, 220
Electronic health records, 12
Etiology, for voice disorders, 159
Evaluation codes, 126
Evaluations. *See* Assessments
Evidence-based evaluations, 82
Examiner effort, 62

F

False negatives, 117
False positives, 117
Fiberoptic endoscopic examination of swallow (FEEs), 179–180
Figurative language, 219
Final reports
 vs. progress reports, **95**
Fluency disorders, 167
 assessment activities for, 171–172
 considerations for assessing, 167–168
 methods for assessing, 169–170
 occurrence of, 168
 wrap-ups for, 172–175
Food, pureed, 179
Formative assessment, 105
Frequency, in voice assessment, 161
Frequency counts, 106
Functional disorders, 159

G

G-Codes, 127
Generalization probes, 109
Glasgow Coma Scale (GCS), 208
Grief, stages of, 21

H

Hard palate, **33**
HCFA 1500 form, 128, **129–130**
HCPCS (Healthcare Common Procedures Coding System) codes, 126
HDHPs (high deductible health plans), 137
 defined, 138
Healthcare Common Procedures Coding System (HCPCS) codes, 126
Health insurance
 activities for, 142–145
 billing methods for, 140–141
 categories of, 137
 definitions of categories, 137–138
 Individual Educational Plans (IEPs) and, 140
 timing of billing for, 139–140
 types of, 137
 wrap-ups for, 145
Health Insurance Portability and Affordability Act (HIPAA) of 1996, 139, 169
 referrals and, 10–11
Health maintenance organizations (HMOs), 137
 defined, 138
Hearing assessment, 115
 activities for, 119–121
 defined, 115–116
 methodology for, 117–118
 purposes of, 116
 screenings for, 116–117
 settings for, 117
 wrap-ups for, 123
Hick picks, 126
High deductible health plans (HDHPs), 137
 defined, 138
High tech, 230
HIPAA. *See* Health Insurance Portability and Affordability Act of 1996
History section, 92
HMOs. *See* Health maintenance organizations (HMOs)

I

ICD-10 CM (International Classification of Diseases, 10th Revision, Clinical Modification) diagnostic codes, 125–126
Identifying Information section, 92
IDs (intellectual disabilities), defined, 207
Independent analysis, of speech sound disorders, 150–151
Individualized Educational Plans (IEPs), 2
 billing for health insurance and, 140
Informal testing, 43
Initial assessments, 19–20
Initial diagnostic assessment reports. *See also* Reports
 defined, 91

Initial diagnostic assessment reports (*continued*)
    sections of, 91–93
        Assessment Information, 92–93
        History, 92
        Identifying Information, 92
        Reason for Referral, 92
        Signature, 93
        Summary and Recommendations, 93
    vs. SOAP notes, **94**
Initial interviews, 19–20
    activities for, 24–26
    clinician behaviors during, 22, **22–23**
    questions asked by clinicians during, 20–221
    reasons for, 21
    settings for, 21
    wrap-ups for, 26–30
Instrumentation measures, 107
Insurance. *See* Health insurance
Intake referral forms
    for adult, 19
    for young child, 19
Intake referral forms, sample, 10, **10**
Intellectual disabilities (IDs), defined, 207
Intelligibility, speech, 152
Intensity, hearing, 117
Interdisciplinary, 187
Interdisciplinary teams, 209
International Classification of Diseases, 10th Revision, Clinical Modification (ICD-10 CM) diagnostic codes, 125–126
Interprofessional collaborative practice (IPCP) teams, 209
IPCP (Interprofessional collaborative practice) teams, 209

J

Jitter, 162
Joint attention, 220

L

Language/literacy
    assessment activities for, 192–197
    authentic component of evaluating, 189
    dynamic assessment and, 188
    evaluation methods for, 189, **190–191**
    reasons for evaluating, 189
    settings for assessment of, 189
    standardized tests for, 188
    timing of screening for, 189
    wrap-ups for, 194–195

Language/literacy assessment, 187–188
    teams for, 187
Language sample analysis, 61
Language samples, 189
Lips, **33**
Listening checks, 117
Literacy. *See* Language/literacy
Low tech, 230

M

Mean, 53
Median, 54
Mediation questions, 63
Medicaid, 137
    defined, 138
Medical referrals, defined, 9
Medicare, 137
    caps on services, 140
    defined, 137
    Part A, 137
    Part B, 137–138
    Part C, 138
    Part D, 138
Modalities, communication, 229
    assessment activities for, 233–235
    wrap-ups for, 235–236
Modifiability Scale, 62
Modified barium swallow study (MBSS), 180
Modified Evans Blue Dye Test, 179
Modifiers, coding, 126
    G-Codes, 127
Motor speech disorders, 149–150
Multidisciplinary teams, 209, 220
Multimodal assessment, 231

N

N, 54
National Provider Identifier (NPI), 9, 138
Neurodegenerative diseases, 208
Neurological syndrome, 197
Noncategorical diagnosis, 187
Nonsymbolic language, 209
Nonverbal skills, 219
Normal bell-shaped curve, 45
Normal developmental disfluency, 167
NPI (National Provider Identifier), 9, 138

O

OASES (Overall Assessment of Speaker's Experience of Stuttering) tool, 170

Objective information, 106–107
  for augmentative and alternative
      communication, 231
Observation, 2, 69, 82
  assessment activities for, 73–75
  components of, 69
  defined, 69–70
  functions of, 70
  methodology, 71–72
  settings for, 71
  specified focus form for, **71–72**
  timing and, 70
  wrap-ups for, 75–78
Ongoing assessments, 2
  activities for, 110–112
  clinical questions addressed using, 107
  introduction to, 105
  reasons for, 107–109
  settings for, 09
  techniques of, 109–110
  timing of, 109
  wrap-ups for, 112–114
Ongoing data, 105
Open focus observation, 71–72
Oral-facial examinations
  activities for, 36–40
  for aphasia assessment, 199
  for dysphagia assessments, 179
  forms available for, 33
  introduction to, 31
  methodology of, 35
  reasons for, 34
  settings for, 35
  timing of, 34
  wrap-ups for, 40–41
Oral peripheral examinations, 160
  defined, 31
  questions to consider when evaluating
      certain oral structures, **32**
  terms for, 31–32
Oral structures, questions to consider when
    evaluating certain, **32**
Organic disorders, 159
Outgoing referral forms, sample, 10, **11**

P

Part-word repetitions, 167
PCC (Percentage of Consonants Correct)
    metric, 152
Penetrating injuries, 207
Percentage of Consonants Correct (PCC)
    metric, 152

Percentages, 106
Percentile rank, 46, 54
Phonotactic inventory, 151
Phonetic inventory, 151
Phonological process errors, 149
PPOs (preferred provider organizations), 137
Practice item, vs. testing item, 44
Pragmatics, 219
Preferred provider organizations (PPOs), 137
  defined, 138
Preliteracy, 187
Pretend play, 220
Primary subscribers, 140
Prior authorization, 139
Probe lists, 108–109
Procedure codes, 126
Prognosis statements, 199
Progress reports, 83, 91
  vs. final reports, **95**
Prolongations, sound, 167
Pureed food, 179

Q

Questionnaires, 82

R

Rancho Los Amigos Levels of Cognitive
    Functioning, 208
Rapid overlapping movements, **33**
Rate, 106
Raw scores, 45, 54
Reason for Referral section, 92
Receptive tasks, 62
Receptive vocabulary, 188
Referrals
  activities for, 13–16
  contents of, 9–10
  format of, 12
  HIPAA and, 10–11
  introduction, 9
  reasons for, 11
  sample completed intake form, **14**
  sample intake form, **10**
  sample outgoing form, **11**
  wrap-ups for, 16–17
Relational analysis, 150–151
Reliability, 54
Reliable information, 84
Reports. *See also* Initial diagnostic assessment
    reports

activities for writing, 98–100
confidentiality and maintenance of, 96
defined, 91–92
methodology for writing, 96–97
purposes of, 93–95
requirements for, 91
"rules" for, 97
timing of, 96
wrap-ups for, 101–103
written, 83
Resonance, 161
Respiration, 161
Right hemisphere syndrome, 197

S

SCDs. *See* Social communication disorders
Scoring, 55
Screening function, 70
Screening requirements, for hearing, 117–118
Screenings, 2
    for aphasia, 199
SD (standard deviation), 45–46, 54
Secondary behaviors, 167
Self-assessment questionnaires, for voice assessment, 160
Self-referrals, 9
Semantic categories, 62
Sensitivity, tests and, 53
Sensorineural hearing loss, 116
Signature section, 93
Silent aspiration, 180
Site of lesion, 197
SLP. *See* Speech-language pathologists
SOAP (Subjective, Objective, Assessment, and Plan) notes, 83, 91, 93, **94**, 105
    vs. Initial Diagnostic Reports, **94**
Social communication, defined, 217
Social communication assessments
    activities for, 221–225
    wrap-ups for, 225–228
Social communication disorders (SCDs)
    assessment methods for, 219–220
    assessment settings for, 219
    authentic assessment, 218
    criteria for, 217–218
    defined, 217
    reasons for assessing, 218
    timing of assessments of, 219
Specific focus observation, 71–72
Specific Intervention, 63
Speech intelligibility, 152
Speech-language pathologists (SLPs), referrals and, 9–11

Speech rate, 170
Speech samples, 169
Speech sound disorders, 149
    activities for, 153–156
    assessment settings for, 151
    designating severity of, 150
    information-gathering methods for, 151–152
    prevalence of, 150
    timing for independent analysis of, 150–151
    types of, 149–150
    wrap-ups for, 157
Spontaneous recovery, 197
Standard deviation (SD), 45–46, 54
Standardized tests/testing, 2, 43
    activities for, 48–49
    administering, 44
    for augmentative and alternative communication, 230–231
    client-appropriate, 43
    as component of assessment, 44
    importance of accurate age and months for giving and scoring, 44–45
    for language/literacy, 188
    process of giving, 43–47
    questions answered by, 43
    reasons for giving, 47
    settings for, 47
    timing of, 47
    wrap-ups for, 49–51
Standard scores, 45
Static assessments, 2
Statistical information, 53
    activities for, 57–58
    settings for clinicians, 55
    terms, 53–55
    wrap-ups for, 58–60
Stimulability testing, 61–62, 151–152
Structured interactions, 2
Stuttering disorders, 167, 168
Subjective information, 106
Subjective, Objective, Assessment, and Plan (SOAP) notes, 93, **94**, 105
    vs. Initial Diagnostic Reports, **94**
Subscriber numbers, 140
Summary and Recommendations section, 93
Superbills, 127, **128**
Swallowing behavior, **33**
Symbolic communications, 209
Synthesizing information, 81–82
    activities for, 85–86
    defined, 82
    methodology, 83–84

reasons for, 82–83
settings for, 83
timing and, 83
wrap-ups for, 87–88

T

TBI. *See* Traumatic brain injury
Team assessment
 for language/literacy, 187
Teeth, **33**
Testing item, vs. practice item, 44
Test manuals, 55
Test-teach-test form, of dynamic assessments, 61–62
Therapy task responses, 107–108
Thresholds, hearing, 118
Tongue, **33**
Tonsils, **33**
Transdisciplinary, 187
Transdisciplinary teams, 209
Traumatic brain injury (TBI), 197, 207–208
 types of
  closed-head injuries, 207–208
  penetrating injuries, 207
Treatment responses, 107–108

U

Unaided/aided help, 230
Unbundled codes, 139

V

Valid information, 84
Validity, defined, 53, 54
Velum, **33**
Verbal reports, 83–84
Video endoscopy, 179
Videofluorographic swallow study (VFSS), 180
Videofluroscopy, 179, 180
Vision loss, 199

Voice assessment, 159
 activities for, 163–164
 defined, 159
 descriptors for, 161
 instrumental options for, 161–162
 methods, 160–162
 reasons for, 160
 screenings for, 160
 settings for, 160
 wrap-ups for, 164–165
Voice disorders, 159

W

Whole-word repetitions, 167
Word finding examinations, 188
Wrap-ups. *See also* Activities
 for adult language assessment, 202–205
 assessment, 5–7
 for billing, 134–135
 for cognitive assessment, 213–215
 for dynamic assessment, 66–68
 for dysphagia assessment, 182–186
 for fluency assessment, 172–175
 for health insurance, 145
 for hearing assessment, 123
 for initial interviews, 26–30
 for language/literacy, 194–195
 for modalities, communication, 235–236
 observation, 75–78
 for ongoing assessment, 112–114
 for oral-facial examinations, 40–41
 referral, 16–17
 for report writing, 101–103
 for social communication assessment, 225–228
 for speech sound disorders, 157
 for standardized tests/testing, 49–51
 for statistical information, 58–60
 for synthesizing information, 87–88
 for voice assessment, 164–165
Written reports. *See* Reports, written